The **Allergy** Book

Sears Parenting Library

The A.D.D. Book
The Attachment Parenting Book
The Autism Book
The Baby Book
The Baby Sleep Book
The Birth Book
The Breastfeeding Book
The Discipline Book
The Family Nutrition Book
The Fussy Baby Book
The Healthiest Kid in the Neighborhood
The Healthy Pregnancy Book
The N.D.D. Book
The Portable Pediatrician
The Pregnancy Book
The Premature Baby Book
The Successful Child
The Vaccine Book

Parenting.com FAQ Books

The First Three Months
How to Get Your Baby to Sleep
Keeping Your Baby Healthy
Feeding the Picky Eater

Sears Children's Library

Baby on the Way
Eat Healthy, Feel Great
What Baby Needs
You Can Go to the Potty

The Allergy Book

*Solving Your Family's Nasal Allergies,
Asthma, Food Sensitivities, and Related Health
and Behavioral Problems*

Robert W. Sears, MD, FAAP, and William Sears, MD, FRCP

Little, Brown and Company
New York Boston London

This book is intended to supplement, not replace, the advice of a trained health professional. If you know or suspect that you have a health problem, you should consult a health professional. The author and publisher specifically disclaim any liability, loss, or risk, personal or otherwise, which is incurred as a consequence, directly or indirectly, of the use and application of any of the contents of this book.

Copyright © 2015 by Robert Sears and William Sears

Little, Brown and Company
Hachette Book Group
1290 Avenue of the Americas, New York, NY 10104
littlebrown.com

First Edition: April 2015

Little, Brown and Company is a division of Hachette Book Group, Inc.
The Little, Brown name and logo are trademarks of Hachette Book Group, Inc.

The publisher is not responsible for websites (or their content) that are not owned by the publisher.

The Hachette Speakers Bureau provides a wide range of authors for speaking events. To find out more, go to hachettespeakersbureau.com or call (866) 376-6591.

ISBN 978-0-316-32480-9
LCCN 2014954181

10 9 8 7 6 5 4 3 2 1

RRD-C

Printed in the United States of America

This book is dedicated to the Sears family children and grandchildren. May you live long, healthy, and allergy-free lives:
Andrew, Annelise, Alex, Joshua,
James, Robert, Peter, Hayden, Erin, Matthew,
Stephen, Lauren, Leah, Jonathan,
RJ, Thomas, Gracie, Sarah, Ashton, Morgan, Landon,
and the newest addition, Levi.

Visit Dr. Bob and Dr. Bill on the Web at www.AskDrSears.com, on Facebook, and at www.DrBobsDaily.com.

Visit www.AskDrSears.com for allergy updates, links to resources, new research, new treatment ideas, conference announcements, and more.

Find us on Facebook at Dr. Bob Sears and Ask Dr. Sears.

And introducing Dr. Bob's new website, www.DrBobsDaily.com, where Dr. Bob shares his daily blog about life inside and outside the office. Enjoy daily updates on parenting, disease prevention, timely news items, humorous anecdotes from his day at work, and inspiring lessons he learns from his patients.

Contents

Authors' Note

This book is intended to provide general information for the treatment of allergies. It is not intended to provide specific medical advice. The treatments presented here are for educational purposes only. If any of the information in this book conflicts with the advice you receive from your own physician, you should follow your physician's instructions. Any medical treatment, whether natural, over-the-counter, or prescription, has the potential to cause harmful side effects. You should seek the advice of your child's primary care physician before beginning any type of treatment for your child.

Introduction

Allergic disorders are the single most common medical and nutritional problem faced by children and adults today. While only a mild nuisance for some, allergies present a lifelong challenge for hundreds of millions of people worldwide. And allergies are more than just a runny nose: they affect virtually every organ system in the body. They irritate the skin, tighten the lungs, inflame the gut, overstimulate or suppress the immune system, and interfere with the proper development and function of the nervous system. Allergies have a profound effect on long-term health and well-being that extends far beyond the annoying symptoms.

The percentage of people who suffer from allergic disorders has steadily risen year after year in recent decades, and this trend shows no signs of slowing. The primary reason for this continued rise is unclear, but most doctors and researchers suspect it is due to environmental influences (chemicals, toxins, pollutants, and poor nutrition) on our genetic health. These influences are compounded by the fact that allergies tend to run in families; parents with allergies have children with allergies, and they grow up to have more allergic children.

This phenomenon is called epigenetics, and it is explained in more detail on page 16. In short, our environment affects how our genes function. Negative environmental influences cause our genes to misbehave and express themselves in unnatural ways. One of these consequences is that the allergic branch of our immune system becomes hyperreactive, and allergic disorders arise. These genetic shifts are passed from parent to child, and the cycle continues. It may be that the best long-term solution to our society's allergy problems is to clean up our planet and our lifestyles. In the meantime, there are numerous steps we can take as individuals to improve our health and alleviate our allergies.

This book was written so that your child won't have to suffer anymore—and neither will you. The course of your life will be changed from one of lifelong symptoms and chronic disease to one of health and happiness. We, Dr. Bob and Dr. Bill, will help you track down what is causing your family's symptoms, and we will tell you how to eliminate the offending agents. For some lucky ones, nothing more is needed. Find the cause and remove it from your life: problem solved. If only it were that simple for everyone. For many, the journey will be more challenging and convoluted. Multiple allergies may be involved. There may be immune dysfunction that needs to be repaired or an inflamed gut that needs to be healed. Treatment may be necessary to bring the body's allergic and inflammatory reactions under control before successful resolution is achieved.

On a personal note, I, Dr. Bob, have suffered from nasal allergies and asthma for most of my life. I have used inhalers on and off (mostly on, until recently). I have been on daily allergy medications. I have used natural supplements. I've been tested for allergies several times. I've tried it all. It has taken years of investigation, but I have finally reached a point where my asthma and allergies no longer affect my daily life, or even my weekly life. I can now go weeks, sometimes months, without turning to my inhaler or pillbox. In the following pages, I will share information about the nutritional and environmental changes I've made and the supplements and natural treatments I use that have made the greatest difference.

A note from Dr. Bob: This book is a collaborative effort between Dr. Bill and me. We share many anecdotes about our experience in the office, and you will notice we refer to ourselves as "we" in such cases. However, as I am the one with allergies, I have more personal stories to share. In the illustrations told from a singular perspective, the "I" refers to me. From here on out, we won't remind you that it's Dr. Bob sharing his life. In the few cases attributed specifically to Dr. Bill, we will make note of that.

Your journey through this book will depend greatly on what type of allergies you and your child have and which of the body's systems are affected. Here is a short preview of each allergic disorder to help you understand the direction in which this book will take you:

Nasal symptoms are perhaps the most common manifestation of allergies. Chronic runny nose, nasal congestion, and sneezing are annoying to both the sufferer and those around them. Careful detective work can likely track down the offending allergens, and, if needed, appropriate testing can reveal the answers. Perhaps it's dust or pets. Maybe it's a food allergy, such as to cow's milk. For those with multiple allergies that cannot be eliminated, appropriate use of allergy medications can bring blessed relief, and natural products are available that can be of equal benefit. Environmental control measures can also reduce exposure to the offending agents. Other causes of nasal problems, such as sinus infections or enlarged adenoids, should be considered when necessary. It is crucial to track down the cause, because those with unresolved nasal allergies are at risk of later developing asthma.

Asthma is a more serious situation that requires treatment beyond allergy testing and the elimination of offending allergens. Medical treatment is usually needed to control asthma symptoms and bring adequate relief to the respiratory system, and it can be safely and effectively administered. Some natural products may also help. But a key aspect of resolving asthma is to reduce the body's inflammation as a whole. The gut must be healed so that the immune system can function appropriately and the allergies and inflammation in the lungs can be relieved.

Skin allergies, such as eczema, hives, and other rashes, are a common occurrence during infancy and can persist through childhood into adulthood. Tracking down and eliminating the causes of skin allergies, and following proper skin care techniques to limit skin irritation, are a must — not only for relief, but also to reduce the risk of asthma.

Food allergies are a growing problem. Some are obvious, such as an immediate allergic reaction to peanuts or shellfish. Understanding how to avoid hidden sources of severely allergic foods is key for those with such allergies. Yet most food allergies aren't so obvious. We will walk you through the investigative steps you should take to determine whether you or your child has food allergies, which foods cause the allergies, and how to maintain proper nutrition as you eliminate those foods from the diet.

Food sensitivities are a whole different ball game. Instead of causing a classic allergic reaction, some foods affect the immune system in a nonallergic way or have a chemical influence on the body and brain. Gluten sensitivity is a growing example, and casein (milk protein) sensitivity is more common than many people believe. Artificial food ingredients take their toll as well.

These effects can manifest themselves as intestinal problems, behavioral challenges, learning difficulties, recurrent illnesses, or even mood disorders.

The medical, behavioral, and developmental conditions that can be attributed to food allergies or sensitivities include infant colic, extreme tantrums, attention and hyperactivity challenges, recurrent ear and sinus infections, autoimmune diseases, and other childhood and adult illnesses. Identifying and eliminating allergies and food sensitivities, and healing the gut and immune system, will improve these conditions.

No matter which bodily system allergies affect, the path to healing should begin by determining which allergens are causing the problem. We provide a complete guide to allergy testing in the following pages, including skin testing, blood testing, and alternative medicine approaches such as muscle testing. But allergy testing isn't perfect, and parents will often need to play allergy detective to determine what their family is allergic to.

Mainstream medicine has come a long way in treating and eliminating allergic disorders. Much of what we share in this book follows the guidelines of the American Academy of Pediatrics, the American Academy of Allergy, Asthma & Immunology, and the American College of Asthma, Allergy & Immunology. We routinely refer patients to pediatric and adult allergists in our area, with great results. But there are times when allergy testing doesn't find the answer and long-term medication isn't ideal for a child. In such cases, an integrative medicine approach is warranted. We will show you how to make appropriate use of natural medicine and alternative medical providers to find the answers you seek. This includes paying close attention to your child's — and family's — nutrition. Hippocrates, the father of medicine, has been quoted as saying, "Let food be your medicine." What you eat can either hurt or help your allergic disorder, so we offer a nutritional plan that decreases body inflammation and allergic reactivity and improves gut and immune health. These steps are essential to successful allergy resolution.

No matter what type of allergies your family has, this book will provide the step-by-step guidance you need to find the appropriate solutions. Our goal is threefold: to help you diagnose your allergies, to help you properly treat your allergies, and, most importantly, to help you eliminate your allergies and improve your long-term health.

The **Allergy** Book

1

The Fascinating World of Allergy and Immunology

We are fascinated by the immune system; the way it interacts with the environment around us is quite extraordinary. But we won't presume that you share the same degree of wonderment that those of us who work in the world of allergy and immunology do. In order to understand allergies, though, you need a general understanding of the immune system. The following section presents a basic overview of how the immune system works, with an emphasis on the allergic branch—and as you read it, you just might find that you too are fascinated.

THE IMMUNE SYSTEM

Allergen is a term you'll see throughout the book, and it refers to anything that triggers an allergic reaction. Our immune system's response to allergens is what causes millions of us to suffer from allergic disorders. Understanding the allergic branch of the immune system will therefore help you understand allergy testing, treatment, and prevention.

The immune system is composed of white blood cells, antibodies, and various chemicals, all of which respond to anything foreign that invades the body. When it comes to germs, white blood cells engulf and kill the germs, then pass the word to the rest of the immune system; this way, the immune system is ready to attack the germ more quickly the next time it comes calling. Cancer cells are eliminated in a similar manner. This type of immunity is a positive thing, as it helps protect us from serious diseases. But when the offending agent is something that triggers an allergic reaction, the response isn't so pleasant.

Our immune system has many different types of white blood cells, each with a unique function, and they all communicate with each other to coordinate their response to invaders. White blood cells are divided into two groups: innate immune cells and adaptive immune cells.

Innate Immunity

Innate immune cells are our first line of defense. These are the sentry cells that immediately attack invaders. Some of these white blood cells, such as natural killer cells and neutrophils, primarily attack germs. Other white blood cells respond to both germs and invading allergens, and include the following:

Mast cells. These are the allergy-responding cells that live in the skin and in our mucous linings (eyes, nose, mouth, lungs, and intestines). They are primarily responsible for releasing histamine when an allergen invades. Histamine is what causes the itching and swelling we experience in an allergic reaction. Mast cells also release chemicals called leukotrienes and cytokines, and certain other acids and enzymes, all of which further the allergic reaction and cause inflammation (redness and swelling).

Basophils. These cells circulate within our bloodstream and release histamine when an allergen enters the bloodstream.

They also release cytokines as part of the body's inflammatory response.

Eosinophils. These cells circulate in the bloodstream and then, when an allergen invades, move into body tissues, where they contribute to the inflammatory response to the allergen. They also attack parasites.

Dendritic cells. These live in our skin and mucous linings. Instead of reacting to the allergens by releasing histamine, as mast cells do, these cells engulf the antigen and bring it to the nearest lymph node, where the antigen is introduced to the *adaptive* part of the immune system (see below). This, in part, is how the rest of the immune system remembers that the body is allergic to that allergen, causing the body to react in the same way to that allergen with each subsequent exposure. Thanks a lot, dendritic cells! These cells aren't all bad, however. They perform the same function with invading germs, so that the body can create better immunity against that germ.

Macrophages. These are another type of "tattletale" white blood cell, which recognize allergens and then send out chemical messages to attract eosinophils, basophils, and some adaptive immune cells.

Epithelial cells. These are actually not white blood cells but structural cells that line the airways of the lungs, bloodstream, and other body tissue linings. These cells respond to allergens by releasing chemicals that attract allergy-fighting white blood cells to the area.

Adaptive Immunity

This branch of the immune system is our second line of defense and is composed of white blood cells called *lymphocytes* and antibodies called immunoglobulins.

Lymphocytes circulate in the bloodstream and congregate in the lymph nodes. These cells, and the antibodies they produce, are the reserves that launch an organized attack on foreign germs and allergens. What sets adaptive immunity apart from innate immunity is memory. When the innate dendritic cells (see above) bring germs and allergens to the lymphocytes, the lymphocytes commit them to memory. On a positive note, this means that the lymphocytes remember past germs and are poised to eliminate those germs when they invade again. Unfortunately, these cells also harbor the memory of what the body is allergic to, and they will launch an allergic response at the slightest provocation. There are two different types of lymphocytes, and each plays a unique role in allergic and immune responses:

1. *T lymphocytes:* These cells kill germs and react to allergens by releasing chemicals called cytokines, which are toxic to the invaders. T lymphocytes provide what is known as cell-mediated immunity, because the immune cells kill invading germs directly. There are several types of T lymphocytes, but two are particularly important in regard to allergies: Th1 cells primarily fight germs and contribute to delayed allergic reactions, whereas Th2 cells are primarily responsible for programming the rest of the immune system to respond to allergens in an allergic manner.
2. *B lymphocytes:* These cells are filled with antibodies that are specific to past germs and allergens. When B lymphocytes encounter those germs and allergens in the blood-

stream, they release the antibodies to attack and destroy the invaders. This process is known as humoral immunity, referring to the bodily fluids, or "humors," which provide the immune response. These cells reside in the mucous lining of body tissues, ready to release their antibodies when an allergen comes along.

Immunoglobulins are the antibodies produced by B lymphocytes. They either float around in the bloodstream or remain within the B lymphocytes, ready to be released when needed. Antibodies neutralize germs and allergens by binding to them. They also help T lymphocytes and other immune cells recognize the invaders. There are five types of antibodies, each with a unique role:

1. *IgM:* This is the antibody that is immediately produced by B lymphocytes in response to an invading germ. It has very little to do with allergies.
2. *IgG:* This is the most prevalent antibody within the bloodstream. It takes longer to produce, but it stays around for a while to continue the cleanup job after the IgM antibodies are used up. IgG antibodies that are specific to past infections will circulate continuously in the bloodstream. It is theorized that IgG antibodies may play a role in chronic allergic responses.
3. *IgA:* This class of antibody circulates in the bloodstream and plays a similar role in germ fighting to those of IgM and IgG. It is also found as a first line of defense where germs tend to invade—namely, in the mucous lining of the nose, mouth, lungs, and gastrointestinal tract. It is present in high levels in breast milk.
4. *IgD:* The role of this antibody is unclear to researchers; it is present in very low levels throughout the body.

5. *IgE:* Last but certainly not least, this antibody class is the bane of allergy sufferers everywhere. It is barely detectable in the bloodstream of healthy individuals, but those with allergies and parasitic infections have high circulating levels. IgE antibodies bind to allergens when they invade the body tissues and initiate the allergic response. You will become intimately acquainted with IgE in the next section and in chapters to come.

THE ALLERGIC IMMUNE SYSTEM

Now you have some general knowledge about how the immune system works. We told you it was fascinating! Next, let's take a closer look at the immune system of a person who suffers from allergies. We guarantee that this will be equally interesting.

Details of the Allergic Response

The first time a person is exposed to an allergen, the dendritic cells bring the allergen to the T lymphocytes in the nearest lymph node. Any potential substance that the person is *not* allergic to is ignored and discarded. But if the lymphocytes recognize the substance as an allergen, a complex cascade of immunological events begins that eventually results in an allergic reaction.

First, the Th2 type of T lymphocytes within that lymph node proliferate in response to the allergen. As you have probably already forgotten, the Th2 lymphocytes are the immune cells primarily responsible for programming the rest of the immune system to react in an allergic manner. They achieve this by secreting cytokines that activate B lymphocytes, the cells that produce the IgE antibodies that will eventually react to that specific allergen the next time it enters the body. This cytokine-mediated activation occurs throughout the body so that B lymphocytes everywhere are primed and loaded with IgE antibodies to be released at a moment's notice. But the cytokines don't stop there. They also program the mast cells, the basophils, and the rest of the innate immune cells that reside in body tissues and mucous linings to be ready to react to that specific allergen.

Enter the allergen for the second time. The IgE antibodies are the first to recognize and bind to the allergen. The innate immune cells then recognize the antibody/allergen complex and respond in two ways: they release various chemicals (histamine, acids, and enzymes), which cause swelling, itching, and irritation in the surrounding tissues, and they release *more* cytokines, which attract more allergy-responding immune cells to the area. T and B lymphocytes are alerted, and the allergic response is propagated throughout the body to varying degrees, depending on how allergic the person is. Histamines also activate sensory nerve cells in the area, which alert the brain to the allergen's presence and help trigger sneezing.

Okay. So how does this translate into the allergic reaction that *you* specifically feel? You can blame that mostly on the histamine. This chemical irritates the body tissues wherever it is released. In the nose, for example, it causes the nasal lining to swell, causes increased mucus production, and provides that wonderful itching sensation. Cytokine chemicals add to the effect. For those of us with asthma, the same thing happens in the airways of our lungs: swelling and mucus. We are spared the itching; instead, we get to experience tight breathing (wheezing) as the muscles that surround our airways respond to the histamine by contracting and squeezing the airways. How about the skin? It's mostly the same process: the redness, swelling, and itching manifest as hives, other rashes, and swelling of entire areas of the body. For those with food allergies, the reaction begins in the lining of the gut, which can result in pain, bloating, and diarrhea.

No matter where the reaction begins, the immune response can spread through the bloodstream to trigger allergic reactions throughout the body. The few who are severely allergic will go into anaphylactic shock; this happens when so many immune cells release their IgE antibodies, histamine, and cytokines simultaneously that severe swelling occurs throughout the body. Blood pressure drops as the blood vessels dilate in response to the histamine, and the person goes into shock.

Chronic Effects of a Heightened Allergic Response

A healthy immune system of a nonallergic person is in perfect balance. With the allergic branch quiet, the germ-fighting, cancer-preventing, and chronic disease–inhibiting aspects of the immune system can do their job. In someone with an allergic disorder, the allergic part of the immune system continues to react as long as the body is exposed to the allergens. The other parts of the immune system are suppressed because the system is expending all of its energy fighting allergies. Furthermore, the overproduction of immune cells and continued release of cytokine chemicals cause ongoing inflammation throughout the body. Chronic allergies can mean more than just annoying symptoms—they can impact lifelong health. We will now introduce you to some key ideas regarding the unbalanced immune system, which we will refer to throughout the book.

Th1/Th2 imbalance. This term describes how the immune system is constantly shifted toward the Th2 side (the allergic branch). The Th2 immune cells actually suppress the Th1 side (the germ-fighting branch)—meaning those with chronic allergies will have low Th1 function, which increases susceptibility to infections. The result is that those with chronic allergic disorders are more prone to have even more problems as they get older. Throughout this book, we stress the importance of finding and eliminating all sources of allergies and focusing on natural ways to keep the Th1/Th2 systems in proper balance.

Persistent class switching. Class switching refers to the ability of the B lymphocytes to switch the class of antibodies they produce. As you learned on page 7, B lymphocytes produce IgA, IgD, IgE, IgM, or IgG antibodies. When a person is fighting an infection, B lymphocytes will switch to producing IgM and IgG. When responding to allergies, they switch to producing the IgE class of antibodies. Those with chronic allergic disorders have a continued switch toward the IgE side. This contributes to the chronic effects of allergies and makes a person more prone to future allergic problems.

Inflammation. We use this term to describe the irritating effects of the cytokines, acids, and enzymes secreted by immune cells. This inflammatory response from the immune system doesn't just occur with allergies. Injuries, infections, chronic diseases, unhealthy foods, and unhealthy lifestyle choices all make the immune system react with an inflammatory response, which damages tissues and causes chronic wear and tear on the body. Eliminating allergic disorders, and following other steps to reduce body inflammation, are crucial for long-term health and wellness.

Autoimmune disorders. These are chronic conditions in which the immune system attacks the body. Diabetes, multiple sclerosis, and lupus are examples in which the immune system turns against a person's own body and attacks a particular organ system. The chronic imbalance of an allergic immune system increases the risk that the immune system is eventually going to turn against the person's own body in an autoimmune manner.

The gut/brain connection. This theory explains why chronic allergies can impact neurological health. The intestinal system is surrounded by nerve cells and nerve centers that regulate gut function. Allergic irritation and inflammation in the gut directly irritate these nerve centers, which, in turn, pass on this inflammation to the central nervous system — the brain. Solving food allergies and sensitivities is critical for long-term neurological health.

The secret to having a healthy immune system and a healthy body is to keep the immune system balanced. This means more than simply taking an allergy pill to reduce your allergy symptoms. That's the easy way out — the pill. We will show you the skills you need to keep the other branches of the immune system in balance so that the allergic branch can rest — and so that you don't need as many pills. The Sears doctors have dubbed this model of health care the Pills and Skills approach, and we refer to it throughout this book.

WHY ARE ALLERGIC DISORDERS ON THE RISE?

Why are allergic disorders becoming more and more prevalent every year? What causes someone to be allergic to something in the first place? Why are some people allergic to something when most others are not? These are intriguing questions — and if we knew the answers, this book would probably be much shorter. We certainly know how allergies happen, how to test for them, and how to treat them. But we don't know many of the reasons why some people have such overactive allergic immune systems. We will present several theories, but the bottom line is that we don't yet know for certain.

We know that genetics plays a significant role in allergic disorders; people with allergies are probably genetically programmed to have them. But what creates that genetic risk in the first place? Here are some hypotheses:

Environmental Toxins

Environmental toxins, such as insecticides, plastics, heavy metals, and pollution, are one reason why allergies may now be more prevalent. Numerous research studies have linked these chemicals to allergic disorders, particularly asthma. These toxins push the immune system over to the Th2 side, which increases inflammation and makes the body more prone to developing allergies. It's not because the person is specifically allergic to those toxins; rather, these toxins make the Th2 lymphocytes much more reactive to common allergens than they should be. Furthermore, toxins damage the body's detoxification mechanisms, rendering the last two generations (us and our children) less able to rid our bodies of the very toxins that are contributing to the problem in the first place.

Genetically Modified Food

Many of the crops we grow, especially corn, soy, and wheat, have been genetically modified or crossbred to resist insects and maximize harvest. Unfortunately, these seemingly minor gene changes alter our food just enough to cause our immune system to view these proteins as foreign invaders instead of food. Most soy used in the United States is genetically modified, and soy is an additive in many foods. In addition, some grain crops have been combined in a way that has increased their allergic potential. Corn, for example, has peanut genes spliced in to enhance growth. And many foods are made with corn syrup as a sweetener, so children are being exposed to peanuts at an early age—and a genetically modified form of peanuts at that. Wheat, the primary grain used by Americans, has been so drastically altered by crossbreeding in recent decades that its current form may cause unwanted allergic and metabolic reactions in many people. Our immune system is more likely to program itself to become allergic to these modified foods. Many countries now ban genetically modified foods, but this is not so in the United States, where food allergies and allergic disorders continue to rise.

Politics and money have a hand in this. Some of our country's major food manufacturers provide significant funding for food allergy research and for organizations that provide food allergy information for families. Such companies and groups downplay the possible link between GMO (genetically modified organism) foods and allergies. Manufacturers are also fighting hard to prevent legislation that would require GMO foods to be clearly labeled; such a law was recently voted down by Californians because it would (supposedly) increase food production costs.

The tide is turning, however. Some states are already changing their labeling laws. And experts estimate that 30 percent of US foods will be non-GMO by the year 2017. One major natural food maker, NOW Foods, pledged to make its entire line of 170 foods completely non-GMO by 2014, and other natural food companies are following suit.

Climate Change

We know it can be fun to blame everything on global warming, but there is some relationship between increasing carbon dioxide emissions and allergies. A recent report in *USA Today* (May 31, 2013) highlighted the science behind this connection. Higher CO_2 levels increase plant growth, and more plants mean more pollen — and voilà, more allergies.

Antibiotic Exposure

It's common knowledge that antibiotics kill the healthy germs in our gut (called intestinal flora or probiotics). These germs play a key role in regulating the immune system in the intestines. Early exposure to antibiotics increases the risk of allergic disorders. Many moms are given antibiotics during labor or during the early months of breastfeeding, which can interfere with an infant's probiotic growth. Add in a few courses of antibiotics during infancy and you set the stage for allergic disorders. In addition, antibiotics are given to cattle and dairy animals, which are then consumed by us and affect our gut flora. Even using antibiotic hand soap has been linked to increased allergies.

Hygiene

There is a theory that our immune system needs to be exercised to remain healthy and balanced. Exposure to germs helps build the immune system. Exposure to some allergens, like pets, helps the allergic branch of the immune system become accustomed to them. Yet parents are more inclined to keep their infants shielded from all germs, especially first-time parents. We don't let our babies crawl on the floor, play outside in the dirt, or touch anything out in public, and we keep disinfectant wipes on hand at all times in case such an infraction occurs. If we try to keep our infants too clean and sheltered, though, we may be doing their immune systems a disservice.

The research isn't conclusive yet, but this theory appears sound. It suggests that we should expose our infants to germs and allergens and not worry so much about keeping everything around them sterile. Sure, you don't want to pick up any germs from sick people, such as in a doctor's office or at the pharmacy counter at a drugstore; but otherwise, kids need some exposure to dirt and germs so that the immune system learns balance.

In our family, perhaps the only thing we still insist on is that the kids wash their hands before dinner. Not breakfast. Not lunch. Just dinner. Old habits die hard.

Epigenetics

This term refers to the study of changes in our gene *function* without physical mutations to the DNA *structure*. Lifestyle, nutrition, stress, medications, diseases, and environmental toxins can actually alter how our genes are expressed, and these changes can be passed on to our offspring. In regard to allergies, we know that if one parent has an allergic disorder, there's a moderate chance that the children will as well. If both parents have allergies, their children are most likely doomed to suffer the same fate. These children are born with the allergic branch of their immune system already revved up, simply due to epigenetically inherited changes in the way their genes control the allergic branch of the immune system.

Methylation Defects

Methylation is a cellular process that turns genes on and off, and some theorize that abnormal methylation function is one reason that the above epigenetic changes are occurring in our population. Methylation is also a key aspect of our detoxification metabolism; if defective, toxins exert even more harm on the immune system. This is important because some integrative medical practitioners are now treating methylation problems to help a variety of medical problems, including allergies. On page 313 we present some ways you can improve your methylation function in order to allow your genes to function better.

CAN ALLERGIES BE PREVENTED IN FAMILIES WITH GENETIC RISK?

Overcoming genetically inherited allergic tendencies isn't easy, but there are numerous steps you can take to lower the risk of allergic disorders in your children. Maintaining a healthy gastrointestinal system is key. Making healthy nutrition and lifestyle choices is also important. And living as green and organically minded as possible may help. The final chapter of this book presents a step-by-step approach to healing and preventing allergic disorders. We hope to learn more in the coming decades that will allow parents to more conclusively reduce inherited allergies in their children.

Given the strong genetic component of allergies, one challenge that allergic families face is deciding whether or not to avoid exposing infants and young children to allergens. Unfortunately, the research is conflicting: Some studies actually show that children who grow up around certain allergens are *less* likely to develop that allergy. It seems they become accustomed to it. For example, children raised around pets or on farms have fewer allergies. Women who eat certain high-allergy foods during pregnancy may be *less* likely to have a child with food allergies. Yet common sense holds that families with such allergies should *avoid* allergens during pregnancy and childhood to reduce the harmful effects of chronic allergen exposure and hopefully reduce the likelihood that the child will develop the same allergy. Research isn't conclusive one way or the other just yet, but the trend seems to be turning toward allowing infants and young children to have some exposure to allergens that run in a family in order to create some tolerance of those allergens. Complete avoidance of family allergens may not be the right choice. Ongoing research will provide better answers in the years to come. We provide prevention advice for specific allergens throughout this book.

2

Allergy Testing

Allergy testing is extremely useful in tracking down the source of allergic disorders. We will provide detailed guidelines on when and how to do allergy testing (and when *not* to do it) for each of the allergic disorders throughout this book. For now, we'll provide a brief overview to facilitate your understanding as you read on.

SKIN TESTING FOR ALLERGIES

This is the traditional and most commonly used method of allergy testing. It is rarely offered by pediatricians or family practitioners; instead, it usually requires a visit to an allergist. The proper name is percutaneous skin testing, but it is more commonly referred to as skin prick or puncture testing. It can be performed at any age.

Procedure

The basic procedure starts with a test solution that contains a particular allergen. A drop of the solution is placed on the skin of the upper back or the inside surface of the forearm. A needle or other sharp device is then passed through the solution into the skin just far enough to puncture the upper layers of the skin, but not deep enough to cause bleeding. This introduces the allergen to the body, and any IgE antibodies that are specific to that allergen, or any innate immune cells that are programmed to react to that allergen, will respond by releasing histamine. This histamine reaction causes the skin to swell and turn red, and the degree of reaction can then be measured in millimeters fifteen or twenty minutes later. The larger the reaction, the higher the allergy. If there is no reaction, the person is not considered significantly allergic to that allergen.

There is a skin test solution for virtually anything a person might wish to test. Numerous allergens can be simultaneously tested, including many foods, animals, pollens, plants, mold, dust, insect venom, and penicillin. The solutions are placed about one inch apart in rows on the skin and labeled for easy reading.

Two control allergen tests are also performed simultaneously. A histamine solution is tested, to make sure the person has reactive skin (virtually everyone shows an allergic skin reaction to histamine). This confirms that the skin testing procedure is valid in that person. A saline skin test (which no one should have a reaction to) is also done as a baseline test to see what a negative reaction looks like on that person.

A more specialized form of skin testing, called intracutaneous or intradermal skin testing, can be done if a person is strongly suspected of having allergies but doesn't react to regular skin testing. It involves injecting the allergen test solution deeper into the skin, which makes it more likely to yield a reaction. But this also has the potential to trigger a severe allergic response, so it is done only when warranted.

The allergen testing solutions used in the United States contain the allergens, saline solution, glycerin, and some electrolytes.

No harmful chemicals or unusual ingredients are used at this time. The test solutions are actually the same products that are used to provide allergy shots (called immunotherapy). See page 264 for more details on these products.

Adverse Reactions to Skin Testing

Skin tests cause little to no pain, but the procedure can be frightening to little children. The cooperativeness of the child should be considered before initiating it. Positive allergic reactions will feel like a mosquito bite and will itch for a day or two. Life-threatening allergic reactions are rare with regular skin prick testing, but emergency medical equipment should be on hand as a precaution. Asthmatics who are currently wheezing should wait until their symptoms are stable to avoid worsening due to allergic response.

Avoiding Allergy Medications Before Testing

The allergist will provide specific guidelines on what to avoid before testing. In general, antihistamine medications should be avoided for about a week beforehand. Some antacids (H2 blocker types) should be skipped on the day of testing. Oral steroids usually don't affect test results. Strong prescription steroid creams can suppress results, though, and should be avoided on the area of skin testing for about three weeks beforehand.

Accuracy of Skin Testing

Skin testing is fairly accurate. If a person is allergic to something, they will very likely have a positive skin test, and a negative skin test is a very reliable indication that the person is not allergic. On the other hand, a positive skin test result may not necessarily mean that the person will experience any noticeable allergic symptoms from that allergen in real life. It is possible for a skin test to trigger a histamine reaction at the site of the test but for the person not to have an allergic reaction when exposed to that allergen naturally. For example, approximately 8 percent of Americans will show an allergic reaction to peanuts on a skin test, but less than 1 percent of Americans are actually allergic to peanuts in real life. We don't yet know why this phenomenon occurs. So if you've had an allergic reaction after eating peanuts, you will probably have a positive skin test. But if you've eaten peanuts numerous times and have had no noticeable reaction, it doesn't really matter what your skin test shows. Skin test results must be correlated with a person's symptoms in daily life. A thorough allergist will consider both when interpreting skin test results.

It is important to know that skin testing for food has value only in determining food *allergies*. It plays no useful role in finding food *sensitivities,* which happen when foods cause behavioral reactions, intestinal discomfort (such as constipation or digestive problems), or autoimmune reactions and immune suppression. A classic example in our practice is when a child has chronic ear infections, intestinal discomfort, hyperactivity, and severe tantrums—or all of the above. The child's skin testing may show no reaction to milk, because the child is not actually allergic; but removing milk products from the diet very often results in improved respiratory, intestinal, and neurological health.

Age is also a factor in the accuracy of both skin and blood testing for allergies. These tests are less likely to register a positive (allergic) result during the first two years of life compared to older children and adults. Testing can and should still be done when needed during infancy, but negative (nonallergic) results don't completely rule out an allergy.

BLOOD TESTING FOR ALLERGIES

This option has grown in popularity as the technology to provide comprehensive and accurate results has improved. Blood testing can be ordered by any doctor, so many pediatricians and family practitioners can use this method without referring patients to an allergy specialist. Virtually everything that can be evaluated through skin testing can be measured through a blood test. Another advantage is that only one needle stick through the skin is needed for the blood to be drawn; however, this may be more frightening for some kids than the lighter prick of skin testing, which can be done out of sight on the child's back. Blood testing is slightly less accurate because a person's allergens are less likely to register as positive on a blood test compared to skin testing. But the positive results that do register are very reliable; whatever shows up as an allergy on the test is accurate. Results are reported on a scale of one through six, with six being highly allergic.

Blood allergy testing can be done via IgE blood testing or IgG blood testing, both of which are outlined below.

IgE Blood Allergy Testing

The mainstream method of blood allergy testing measures IgE levels for various allergens. As you read in Chapter 1, an allergic person will have IgE antibodies circulating in the bloodstream that are specific to that person's allergies. There are two basic panels of tests that can be ordered by doctors. The first is a food panel, which measures the most commonly allergic foods, like eggs, milk, wheat, tree nuts, peanuts, fish, and soy. Many other foods can be added to the testing as well. The second is an inhalant panel, which measures airborne allergens like pollen (from plants and trees), animals, dust, mold, and other environmental allergens. Inhalant panels are usually region-specific; they measure the pollens that are known to occur in that area of the country. Cockroach infestation can also cause allergies, and this can be tested in the blood for those who live or work where cockroaches thrive. Doctors commonly order both food and inhalant panels when evaluating allergies. We often start with blood allergy tests for our patients and then refer them to an allergy specialist for skin testing if the blood result doesn't find the answers.

IgG Food Sensitivity Blood Testing

In addition to IgE levels, a growing number of integrative medical doctors are ordering blood panels to measure IgG levels for a large number of foods. IgG antibodies are the type of immunoglobulins that B lymphocytes generate primarily to fight infections. Yet these cells also create IgG against almost anything foreign that is found in the bloodstream. The presence of IgG antibodies against foods indicates that the immune system is reacting against those foods.

The significance of this immune reaction is not yet known. Very little research on IgG food testing exists, and the FDA and most medical organizations do not recognize IgG reactions as valid indications that such foods cause any problems. But many physicians who practice alternative medicine believe that high levels of IgG antibodies to foods do indicate that a person is sensitive to those foods.

These test results are often used as a guide for elimination diets to help heal the gut and immune system and improve various chronic symptoms such as fatigue, headaches, lack of focus, hyperactivity, recurrent illnesses, and neurodevelopmental disorders. Some research supports the usefulness of IgG food results as an elimination diet guide to alleviate migraine headaches, but very little research exists for other health problems, including allergic disorders. Some laboratory companies also test

IgM and IgA food antibodies along with IgG, to measure the entire immune system's response to foods. But there is no evidence that this three-pronged approach increases the accuracy or usefulness of these tests.

There are several aspects of the IgG/food theory that it is important to understand:

The IgG/food theory holds that the chronic elevation of IgG from food overstimulates the immune system and contributes to body inflammation. While the immune system is busy fighting these foods, other branches of the system are dysfunctional or suppressed. Theoretically, removing such foods from the diet would allow the immune system to calm down, thus reducing inflammation throughout the body.

We don't yet know why some people react to foods in this manner. With classic IgE, we know that the allergy is programmed into the person's genes. But we don't know whether this is true for people with IgG reactions. Some theorize that people might react because they eat too much of a certain food; others believe that the reaction does indicate an inherent sensitivity, even to small amounts of the food. Still others believe that the leaky gut theory better explains these IgG reactions.

The leaky gut theory is an emerging idea in medicine that may partly explain these sensitivities; the medical term is *increased intestinal permeability*. The intestinal lining is made up of tightly packed cells that are designed to absorb digested nutrients, process them, then pass them through to the bloodstream as amino acids, sugars, fats, and vitamins and minerals for the rest of the body to enjoy. This lining is supposed to be *impermeable* to almost everything else. Unfortunately, intestinal irritation (from allergenic foods, infections, unhealthy inflammatory foods, and other factors) causes the bond between intestinal cells to loosen, creating a space between them through which anything can "leak." This means that large proteins from partly digested foods can leak into the bloodstream; the immune system then recognizes these large food proteins as foreign invaders and creates an IgG immune response to them. This is what is measured in an IgG food panel.

It is theorized that those with multiple food IgG sensitivities (twenty or more) probably have a leaky gut that is allowing the many incompletely digested food proteins into the bloodstream. And this is a vicious cycle: the foods inflame the immune system, which worsens intestinal irritation, which makes the leaky gut even leakier. The person may not actually be inherently sensitive to these foods, as those with genetically programmed IgE food allergies are. Rather, it is the leaky gut phenomenon that creates the sensitivities. The cycle continues until the gut is healed, the large food proteins no longer leak through, and the immune system calms down.

Those who show only a few IgG reactions on their food panel probably don't have a leaky gut; these few foods may be irritating the immune system and contributing to chronic symptoms, but the gut itself may be in good shape.

It is believed that eliminating the IgG-reactive foods from the diet for several months helps the immune system and the gut to heal, especially if there are many reactive foods on the test result. Other measures to improve intestinal health, such as anti-inflammatory diets and gut-healing supplements (detailed in Chapter 14) may also help heal the leaky gut and reduce the food-induced immune irritation.

We believe this complicated theory has merit, but it is not yet backed up by sufficient research to make it fact. Nonetheless, fixing a leaky gut is an important step in healing body inflammation, multiple food allergies and sensitivities, and other allergic disorders. In Chapter 14 we explore how to achieve this.

As an integrative medical practitioner, I have used IgG food testing in many patients. In some cases, I have found the elimination of positive foods useful in improving health. But I fully acknowledge the current lack of adequate research into the success rate of these tests. Another drawback of these tests is the cost. Costs can range between $100 and $600—or more—and medical insurance often doesn't cover it. Throughout this book we discuss which circumstances warrant consideration of IgG food testing.

A final note on IgG testing: If you are going to do testing, you must do so before eliminating any foods. Once a food is eliminated from the diet for a few weeks, IgG tests will be less likely to register a sensitivity to it, so the test won't be useful.

COMBINING SKIN AND BLOOD TESTING

Skin and blood allergy tests often yield different results, especially in children under four. One method may miss allergies that the other will pick up. If allergy elimination based on one test doesn't result in resolution of symptoms, consider testing with the other method to uncover more allergies.

ALTERNATIVE ALLERGY TESTING TECHNIQUES

Muscle strength testing has become the most popular method of alternative medical testing for allergies. Some of our family members have tried it. We are very open-minded physicians, and we use many alternative medical approaches in our practice. But we just can't seem to wrap our mainstream medically trained minds around this particular method.

The muscle strength testing process involves placing the suspected allergic substance in the patient's hand, then pushing down on the arm. If the person is sensitive or allergic, the arm will be weaker. We have also seen this test performed by placing the allergens on the chest or abdomen and testing arm strength.

A variation of this method involves measuring electrical impulses through the body while a person is touching suspected allergens.

Sounds a bit crazy, right? Well, we have had hundreds of adult patients tell us that such methods have been spot-on in pinpointing their allergies. Our office has seen many infants and children with colic or food allergies who have had success when this method has been used by alternative health care practitioners. Anecdotally, it seems to work. But it would be helpful if at least one peer-reviewed medical research study could verify it.

An extension of muscle testing for allergies is a technique called NAET, in which the goal is to actually eliminate the allergies — to make the body no longer allergic to that substance. Nambudripad's Allergy Elimination Technique was developed by Dr. Devi Nambudripad, a medical doctor with training in acupuncture and chiropractic. It combines applied kinesiology, acupuncture, acupressure, and chiropractic methods to eliminate allergies. NAET has very little medical research to support it, and every mainstream American medical association discounts it. I have not (yet) tried it for my own allergies, but I am certainly curious to hear and see more. If I ever get around to trying it, I'll let you know on DrBobsDaily.com.

No type of allergy testing is completely reliable, and test results should never be the ultimate factor in your allergy decisions. The most accurate indicator of an allergy is to observe a person's reaction to a suspected allergen. Testing is a useful tool that helps in many situations, and we will provide insights on how you should use and interpret skin test results for each allergic disorder that we discuss throughout this book.

3

Nasal and Eye Allergies

Nasal allergy is the most common manifestation of allergic disorders, affecting about 20 percent of Americans. The medical term is *allergic rhinitis,* but we'll keep it simple by calling it nasal allergy. These allergies can occur at any age, although they most commonly begin around ten years of age.

Ocular (eye) allergies often accompany nasal allergies. Some people, on the other hand, *only* have ocular allergies. The two have similar causes and similar treatments. In this chapter, we focus much of our discussion on nasal allergies. At the end, we present eye-specific details for those of you who suffer only from ocular symptoms.

I have suffered from nasal allergies ever since junior high. I remember filling my pockets with toilet paper so I could blow my nose every hour at school...all day long...every day. This went on for years. Some seasons were better than others, and I'd occasionally have some allergy-free months. But I was pretty miserable during flare-ups. I didn't take any allergy meds, and it never even occurred to me to ask my parents for help. I just suffered through it.

I've since discovered through skin allergy testing that I'm seriously allergic to dust, am mildly allergic to mold, and have some pollen allergies. I still have some allergy days every year, but they are few and far between. Dust-prevention steps in my home and office have played a key role in this. Following some antiallergy nutritional guidelines, as outlined in Chapter 14, has also helped. I've also tried some natural allergy supplements (homeopathic oral sprays for dust and regional pollens, as well as quercetin) with good results. Currently, I only have to pop an allergy med about ten random days each year. I sneeze a few times each day, but I no longer suffer from an itchy, runny nose or persistent sneezing the way I used to. During the writing of this book, I spent an entire afternoon sorting through boxes of old papers and books, an endeavor that would normally have had me sneezing within minutes. To my pleasant surprise, I didn't experience even a single sneeze or drip. It seems as if my nutritional and lifestyle changes have minimized my dust allergy. I hope those of you who suffer from nasal allergies are encouraged by this story. Now let's work together to solve *your* family's nasal allergies.

A CLOSER LOOK AT THE ALLERGIC IMMUNE SYSTEM IN THE NOSE

Remember the fascinating immunology you learned in Chapter 1? We know you're itching to learn more, so we'll explain what happens in the nasal passages of those with nasal allergies:

An allergen particle, such as a speck of pollen or dust, enters the nose and sticks to the mucous lining (or more accurately, hundreds of such particles enter at the same time). IgE antibodies, which have already been programmed by the immune system to react to that allergen from past exposures, attach to it. The activated IgE then attaches to nearby mast cells, which causes the cells to release their histamine and other chemicals. These chemicals cause the mucous lining to swell, trigger more mucus secretion, and prompt blood vessels in the nose to leak fluids into the area. Sensory nerves within the nose are also activated by histamine, which triggers sneezing. More white blood cells, such as eosinophils, are drawn in to secrete more inflammatory chemicals. The result is an itching, sneezing, runny nose and nasal congestion, and the process continues as long as the allergens continue to enter the nose.

HOW TO DETERMINE WHETHER YOU OR YOUR CHILD HAS NASAL ALLERGIES

Nasal allergies are usually obvious: the persistently itchy, runny nose and recurrent sneezing are a dead giveaway. Timing patterns are also a clue; look for symptoms that last longer than you'd expect for a common cold (a few weeks), symptoms that randomly occur on windy days without progressing into an illness, or symptoms that predictably flare up during certain seasons of the year. But sometimes it's not so clear. Subtler clues to nasal allergies include the following:

- An allergic crease (a horizontal line above the tip of the nose where the skin folds when a child rubs the itchy nose)
- Itching of surrounding areas (palate, ears, eyes)
- Plugged ears and sinuses without feeling sick
- Clear nasal mucus (as opposed to the thicker mucus associated with illness)
- Chronic sore throat and/or cough without feeling ill
- Location of symptoms (symptoms at home but not at school, or vice versa, or symptoms only at night in the bedroom)
- Chronic fatigue, headache, or irritability
- Recurrent sinus infections or cold symptoms that become chronic

To put it simply, allergies are itchy, sneezy, and drippy; illnesses are thick, stuffy, and droopy (meaning, your child feels ill).

Parents in our office often wonder whether their child's cough and cold symptoms could be allergies. Our quick answer? It doesn't matter…at least not yet. The simplest approach is to treat the symptoms with OTC cold and allergy meds (or some natural treatments) to give your child some relief (see "Treating Nasal Allergies," page 40). If it's a cold, it will pass within a few weeks. If it progresses into a sinus infection, you'll see a sinus headache, thick nasal secretions, facial pain, and persistent fever. If it's an allergy, it may be gone in a day or two (if it's simply an allergy day due to high pollen count), or it may persist for weeks or months without progressing into other symptoms of illness.

A common misconception is that a doctor can examine a child and determine for sure whether it's allergies, a common cold, a sinus infection, or something else. While some classic textbook signs indicate allergies versus illness, these aren't predictable or reliable enough for a doctor to be certain from an office visit. Ultimately, observing the pattern and duration of symptoms, along with a physical exam, provides the most accurate indicators. There are some other causes of a chronic runny nose and congestion that your doctor can rule out on physical examination. These include sinus infection, enlarged adenoids, foreign body, and nasal polyps. When these are ruled out and the pattern of symptoms has declared itself as allergies, it's time to go to work to track down the cause.

CAUSES OF NASAL ALLERGY

While nasal allergies can be triggered by pretty much any allergen, some allergens more commonly trigger allergic responses within the nose. These include:

- Pollen
- Mold
- Dust
- Pets
- Cockroaches
- Cow's milk

One or more of these six items is the most likely trigger of nasal allergies (as well as of asthma, which we will explore in Chapter 4). Other causes are possible, but these are the ones that are worth focusing on first. I happen to be mostly allergic to dust, and somewhat to mold, with some seasonal pollens thrown in. I'm fine with all animals and cow's milk, and cockroaches don't bother me at all. Well, I should say they don't bother my immune system; I'll be the first one to jump up onto a kitchen chair, screaming, if I see one scamper across the kitchen floor.

IS IT ALLERGIES? LET A PILL DECIDE.

When in doubt, one useful way we've found to determine whether someone has allergies or just a prolonged cold is to try an allergy med for three days. If symptoms improve, you know it's allergies. You then stop the med and begin investigating. See page 41 for medication choices.

TRACKING DOWN THE CAUSE OF NASAL ALLERGIES

Now that you've determined that you or your child has nasal allergies, where do you start your investigation to figure out the cause? Here's a simple step-by-step approach we use in the office every day. It begins by considering the age of the child.

Infants with Nasal Allergies

Classic nasal allergies due to dust, mold, and pollen usually don't begin until later in childhood. Infant immune systems rarely become sensitized to these allergens, so they typically don't play a role in infant allergies. The most common cause of infant nasal allergies, by far, is cow's milk. This can occur when the cow's milk proteins in a mom's diet transfer through the breast milk or when an infant is fed a cow's milk–based formula. In practice, infants who are sensitive to cow's milk will likely have many more symptoms than simple nasal congestion; gastrointestinal problems, skin reactions, and other respiratory symptoms will likely accompany the nasal congestion if the allergy is severe. In fact, these other manifestations of allergies are usually more severe than the nasal symptoms. But mild milk allergy can cause nasal symptoms alone. We explore cow's milk allergy in more detail in Chapter 7, Milk Allergy and Sensitivity. But it's worth an early mention now, because eliminating cow's milk from the equation is an important first step in resolving infant allergies. If you've eliminated cow's milk for several weeks without results, consider a soy allergy; this is another common cause, and soy can also be passed through the breast milk or infant formula.

Be sure to consider irritants in the air, such as perfumes or scented body lotions, household cleaning products, and cigarette smoke. We can't tell you how many times we've found that Grandma's heavy perfume is the cause of a baby's wheezing and congestion. Even some facial makeups emit a heavy, irritating scent.

If nasal symptoms persist despite these changes, consider other foods in Mom's diet or the type of infant formula. Perhaps it's a family pet. Dust allergy is uncommon at a young age, but possible. If you and your doctor still can't figure it out, it may be time for allergy testing, especially if the nasal allergy is accompanied by other allergies in other body systems. The decision to do blood allergy or skin allergy testing should be made on a case-by-case basis. If testing reveals some allergens, you eliminate those from the infant's life. See Chapter 13 for instructions on eliminating specific inhalant allergens. Chapter 6 explores food allergy symptoms and testing during infancy in more detail, and the chapters that follow discuss specific food allergies.

However, it's important to know that infant immune systems don't always register allergic responses on allergy tests. Allergy results for infants are useful when they show an allergy, but they don't rule out allergies with negative results. An infant could be allergic to cats, for example, but have completely normal test results. If your allergy testing doesn't yield any answers, and you've removed cow's milk from the baby's life without improvement, your next step is to reduce exposure to the most common airborne allergens, like dust, mold, pollen, and pets. Make the bedroom as dust-free as possible. Inspect the home for mold. Keep the family pet out of the bedroom during the day and night. Follow pollen-prevention measures. Chapter 13 provides details on each of these steps.

Toddlers/Preschoolers with Nasal Allergies

Between one and four years of age, cow's milk is still the most likely cause of nasal allergies, and a milk-free diet is your best first step (see page 138). This is especially true if the chronic nasal symptoms are accompanied by recurrent ear and sinus infections. A common scenario in our office is the fifteen-month-old who has been drinking whole cow's milk since his first birthday, and lo and behold, he has had a chronic runny nose ever since. Any such child deserves a milk-free trial period, and for more than half of you reading this section, your job as allergy detective stops here. But some of you will need to continue the investigation into household and outdoor allergens. Blood or skin testing becomes more accurate the older the child gets, and it's a useful option at this young age if symptoms are problematic.

However, you may be able to figure out what's causing your child's allergies without resorting to testing. In the next section, we show you how to be a successful allergy detective.

COULD IT BE THE ADENOIDS?

Adenoids are synonymous with the tonsils, but they sit in the back of the nose instead of the throat. They can enlarge during the preschool and elementary years and cause chronic nasal obstruction. The primary sign of adenoid enlargement is obstructed nasal breathing; affected children will breathe through the mouth to compensate. Those with enlarged adenoids may *think* they are chronically congested from allergies — and may waste many months or years chasing down allergies — when in fact it's simply a structural problem. The most common cause of enlarged adenoids is recurrent sinus infection; frequent colds can also be a cause, and some will experience adenoid enlargement for no particular reason at all. The challenge is that the adenoids can remain large for many years. They can also become chronically infected, and can be a source of sinus infection themselves. The resulting chronic nasal congestion, obstructed breathing, and recurrent sinus infections take their toll on a child's well-being. A primary care doctor cannot visualize the adenoids because they are too far back in the nose to see. Adenoid enlargement is diagnosed either by X-ray or upon examination by an ear, nose, and throat specialist (ENT). Your primary care physician will help you decide the right course of action.

In some people, enlarged adenoids can be caused by allergies, so treating and solving the allergies should bring relief *if* allergies are the culprit. If a child has many of the nasal allergy symptoms described on page 30, particularly an itchy, runny nose, sneezing, *and* chronic nasal obstruction, it may be allergy-based adenoid enlargement. If congestion is the *only* symptom, without a clear runny nose, itching, and sneezing, it's likely nonallergic.

Nasal Allergies in Older Children and Adults

As children get older, nasal allergies become more common, often manifesting around ten years of age. Some kids will enjoy an allergy-free childhood, then begin the sneezing and runny nose as they grow and their immune system changes. Milk allergy is unlikely to develop at this later age, as it would have presented during the first years; the same goes for other food allergies. If, on the other hand, you think back and realize that this problem dates to toddlerhood, a milk-free trial is a must before you go any further.

Late-onset nasal allergies are more likely due to environmental triggers than to foods. Testing will be of great value in tracking down the allergens, but you can play detective before jumping into testing. Here's how:

Year-round symptoms. Those who are allergic all year long are most commonly allergic to dust, cockroaches, animals, or foods.

Nighttime symptoms only. If your child is generally well all day, but the sneezing, congestion, and coughing occur during the night, it's obvious your child is allergic to something in the bedroom. That "something" is most likely dust, as bedrooms are the dustiest part of the house. Dust-proof the bedroom and see if your child improves. Also inspect the bedroom for mold, as mold is another possibility. If the family dog loves to curl up on your child's bed day or night, this will increase nighttime symptoms if your child is allergic. Keep the family pet out of the bedroom for a few weeks to see if nighttime symptoms improve. Chapter 13 provides further details on how to eliminate dust, mold, and other inhalant allergies.

Seasonal symptoms. If your family is allergic only during certain seasons, with months of wellness during much of the year, a pollen allergy is most likely. Trees primarily pollinate in the late winter into spring, grass in the late spring into summer, and weeds in the late summer into fall. Children who are allergic to only one of these groups of plants will have allergy symptoms during that season. A child may be allergic to two or three of the groups, in which case you will see allergies for months at a time, with some months "off" during the late fall, winter, and mid-summer. It's impractical to expect you to successfully avoid all exposure to pollens in a child who is essentially allergic to the outdoors, but on page 261 you will find some practical ways to at least reduce the amount of pollen your child inhales during these seasons. Certain molds also have a seasonal pattern, of which you should be aware (see page 255).

Blustery days. If symptoms seem to flare on windy days, pollen allergy is the most likely trigger, and maximizing your pollen-preventing efforts on those days can help. Mold spores will also blow around in the wind.

Rainy days. Household mold thrives during wet weather. If your symptoms worsen on rainy days, you may be reacting to areas of mold within the home. On page 255, you will investigate how to find and eliminate mold.

Combined eye and nasal allergies. Pollen allergies tend to trigger ocular symptoms in addition to nasal symptoms. This combination is a clue to pollen as the cause, especially if both eyes are affected and symptoms are seasonal.

School-related symptoms. Children who are well at home but complain of allergies at school may be allergic to a classroom pet or a particular pollen blooming nearby. Cockroach allergy is another possible factor. These children may also be sensitive to the harsher industrial cleaning agents used at school or the off-gassing of chemicals from building materials in a newly built or renovated classroom. A classroom change for medical reasons may be warranted.

Work-related symptoms. Those with symptoms only at work should consider the above factors as well. Cockroach allergy is a likely possibility for those who work in food production, warehouses, or storage facilities. See page 259 for details.

Heating/air-conditioning ducts. Some people will have allergic responses to dust and mold coming out of a central heating or air-conditioning system. Notice whether or not symptoms are related to the time of year or time of day when your system is in use. A good duct cleaning and the installment of proper filters can fix the problem (see page 252).

If you or your child fits well into one of the above patterns, you may find relief by focusing your energy on limiting exposure to suspected allergens. In Chapter 13, you will find detailed instructions on how to eliminate various inhalant allergens from your family's life. If you don't find relief, testing is the next step. Your pediatrician or family doctor can help you decide whether blood testing is the best option, or whether a visit to an allergy specialist for skin testing is warranted.

NONALLERGIC RHINITIS

Not all runny noses are caused by allergies or the common cold. There is a condition called nonallergic rhinitis; this refers to those with chronic runny noses that are not a result of a classic IgE allergic immune reaction to an allergen. Consider the following reasons for your child's runny nose before you assume that allergies are the cause:

Vasomotor rhinitis. This type of runny nose occurs due to dilation of nasal blood vessels and increased nasal mucus caused by environmental factors and irritants other than allergens. Triggers include temperature or humidity changes; exposure to irritants like perfumes, smoke, and cleaning agents; chlorine from swimming pools; exercise; and even emotional changes.

Gustatory rhinitis. This refers to runny nose due to physiologic reactions to spicy foods, hot foods, and even alcohol.

Medication-induced rhinitis. Certain drugs can trigger runny nose as a side effect, including aspirin, ibuprofen, and other non-steroidal anti-inflammatory medications; oral contraceptives; and blood pressure and cardiac meds. Be aware that using OTC decongestant nasal sprays for more than three to five days can cause a rebound effect; nasal congestion can actually increase when the med is stopped.

Hormonal rhinitis. Hormonal changes that occur during puberty, menstruation, pregnancy, and lactation, and with thyroid disease, can trigger nasal symptoms. Increased blood volume during pregnancy can increase nasal blood flow and congestion.

Work-related exposures. Some occupations expose people to airborne irritants, both allergic and nonallergic. People in these occupations include farmers and livestock caretakers, veterinarians, workers in food processing plants, workers who assemble electronic equipment, and laboratory workers.

TREATING NASAL ALLERGIES

Eliminating specific allergens is the most important step in allergy treatment. This is easy when the allergen is something you *can* eliminate, such as a particular food. But many of us are allergic to things that are impossible to get rid of completely. Dust is everywhere. Pollen permeates the air outside. Pets are often integral members of the family. For these allergens, the best we can do is *reduce* our exposure. Some of these allergens are going to find their way into our mucous linings and trigger allergic responses, and periodic treatment will be necessary. For some, chronic treatment may be needed. There are some safe and effective over-the-counter and prescription allergy meds to choose from, and various natural treatments also work well. For those with severe, persistent nasal allergies, allergy shots can help. And, of course, don't forget to incorporate proper allergy-preventing nutrition for your family (page 289).

Home Measures

In our Pills and Skills model of health care, introduced on page 12, taking allergy pills may be easy, but it isn't an ideal long-term solution. Following some natural daily measures to reduce nasal symptoms takes a little more skill but is worth the effort.

Hose the nose. Flushing the pollen, dust, pet dander, and other allergens out of the nasal mucosa on a daily basis, or even twice daily, with saline can reduce the degree of allergic reaction. Gently rinse the nose out with a plastic nasal saline bottle (available at any drugstore), but be careful how aggressively you rinse; high-pressure sprays of saline can irritate the nose and ears. Even more effective, and gentler, is a neti pot, which rinses saline through the nose without using pressure. For children who won't tolerate these, a gentle saline mist spray, followed by a nose blow, can be effective enough. When I feel a nasal allergy attack coming on, a quick trip to the bathroom for a saline rinse is sometimes all I need—no pill required. You can buy nasal saline or make your own by dissolving a quarter teaspoon of salt in eight ounces of water.

Steam clean. For children who resist nasal saline, a good steaming can be of some benefit. Ten minutes in a steamy shower or bathroom, breathing through the nose and blowing several times, cleans out allergens. A facial steamer is also useful for older kids.

Over-the-Counter Antihistamines

These medications are the mainstay of allergy treatment. I have found them extremely effective in giving me allergy-free days when I need them. Side effects are virtually nonexistent. Antihistamines work by binding to what are called the H1 receptors on the white blood cells, blood vessel lining, mucus-secreting cells, and sensory nerve cells. These H1 receptors are where histamine chemicals (released during the initial phase of an allergic reaction) bind to further activate the allergic response. But antihistamine medications bind to these receptors instead and render them inactive for several hours or more. So when an allergen enters the nose and histamine is released by the local immune cells, the histamine can't continue the allergic response by binding to any receptors in the area. There are several OTC antihistamines to choose from:

Short-acting, sedating antihistamines. Diphenhydramine (known by the brand name Benadryl) is a reliable medication that works very well for almost any allergic reaction. It is an ingredient in many OTC cold and allergy preparations, sometimes combined with other cough and cold ingredients. This is a fine choice for spur-of-the-moment use, and we recommend using a dye-free formulation (generic brand is fine). It causes drowsiness in most people and hyperactivity in a few, and it only lasts four to six hours, so it isn't a proper choice for routine use. It can cause oversedation in infants, so check with your doctor before using with children under one year of age. Chlorpheniramine is a similar medication that can also be used.

Long-acting, nondrowsy antihistamines. Fexofenadine (brand name Allegra), cetirizine (Zyrtec), and loratadine (Claritin) are the three most commonly recommended OTC antihistamines. They are long-acting (twelve to twenty-four hours) and do not cause drowsiness. I use fexofenadine when I need an antihistamine. Some of these antihistamines are available as liquids or melt-in-the-mouth tablets, so they are easy to use on young children. These meds began as prescription, then became OTC as their safety and ease of use were proven. We recommend one of these three choices for anyone who requires a medication for allergies, whether it's occasional one-time use or routine daily use. These meds are also available OTC in combination with a decongestant, labeled as the drug name with a *D* after it, for those with allergies in whom nasal congestion is a problematic factor.

Over-the-Counter Nasal Sprays

Most allergy nasal sprays are prescription, but there are two types that are OTC:

Cromolyn (brand name Nasalcrom). This medication is a mast cell stabilizer, meaning it prevents the mast cells from releasing their histamine. It doesn't work well as a quick-relief antihistamine. Instead, it is designed for ongoing use as prevention against nasal allergy flare-ups.

Steroids. Until now, these have always been prescription. The FDA has just approved low-dose formulations for OTC use. Nasacort is the first to become available, and others are likely to follow soon. See below for more information.

Prescription Medications

When stronger treatment is necessary, there are several forms of prescription meds to choose from: oral antihistamines and steroid nasal sprays are the most commonly used, and oral leukotriene inhibitors and antihistamine nasal sprays are also worthy options.

Long-acting, nondrowsy oral antihistamines. Two of these meds (desloratadine and levocetirizine) are upgraded versions of their OTC counterparts. They aren't necessarily much better; they are simply newer and still require a prescription. They will likely be OTC in the coming years. We've had no experience with these meds so far, as we've found the OTC versions effective. There are other prescription antihistamines that allergy specialists may choose that are beyond the scope of this book.

Steroid nasal sprays. These are a favorite med among allergists. They work by inhibiting various white blood cells' response to allergens. There are too many choices to list here, and we have no preference for one over any other. We know that most parents are hesitant to give their child any type of medical steroid treatment on an ongoing basis. A common worry regarding steroid treatments is that they may stunt growth in children. A recent study of 180 children ages five to eight who used a steroid nasal spray for one year showed just a quarter-centimeter less growth compared to 180 children who did not use a steroid. Because the effect on growth is minimal, we do prescribe these from time to time for patients who have severe nasal allergies and congestion that don't respond to oral antihistamines and other measures.

Antihistamine nasal sprays. These are a good option for people who are not comfortable with nasal steroids. Efficacy isn't quite as reliable, but when these sprays are successful, they are preferable to chronic steroids.

Oral leukotriene inhibitors. This class of medication is a fairly recent development. Montelukast (brand name Singulair) is the best known. Instead of blocking the histamine receptors, this med attaches to the receptors that leukotrienes (inflammatory chemicals similar to histamine) bind to, preventing activation of part of the allergy response. This med is also used in asthma treatment.

Deciding When and How to Treat with a Medication

Ultimately, your doctor should help you create an allergy treatment plan for you or your child. It's likely that your plan will require pills for allergy treatment from time to time. As an allergy sufferer myself, and having suffered from untreated symptoms as a child, I know firsthand the relief that allergy medications can bring. Here are some guidelines we follow in our office for using allergy medications:

Occasional symptoms. For random allergic days here and there, an OTC long-acting, nondrowsy oral antihistamine is a good choice. If this doesn't work well, your doctor may provide you with a prescription version.

Occasional nighttime symptoms. You may find a short-acting, sedating OTC antihistamine a good choice for occasional nighttime symptoms. If, however, you find that bothersome symptoms have returned by morning, you may need the long-acting OTC version above.

Prolonged symptoms that are seasonal. If you predict that the allergies are going to continue daily through spring or fall, first try an OTC long-acting, nondrowsy oral antihistamine. If that's not enough, try either a prescription version or a nasal spray. If neither choice is adequate, try using both simultaneously for a week or two. When the season is over, stop the meds.

Year-round allergies. If everyday treatment is needed on an ongoing basis, an antihistamine nasal spray may be the best choice, if it is effective enough. A steroid nasal spray may be a good second choice, or consider an oral leukotriene inhibitor. Long-acting, nondrowsy antihistamines can also be used chronically. But if your allergies are this persistent, dedicate more time to pursuing preventive and diagnostic measures, and explore natural treatment options that are safer for long-term use.

Flare-up of severe congestion and headache. If sinus symptoms worsen during allergy flare-ups, add an OTC decongestant to your allergy medication (or use a *D* version of your current antihistamine; see page 42) and step up the nose-hose and steam clean sessions.

Allergy Shots

Many people naturally shy away from allergy shots. But we encourage patients to consider this therapy under the right circumstances. Known by the medical community as immunotherapy, allergy shots can literally remove a person's allergic tendencies toward a variety of allergens, including pollens (grass, ragweed, and others), dust mites, cats, dogs, cockroaches, and some molds. See page 264 for a detailed discussion on allergy shots.

Two particularly exciting aspects of immunotherapy are emerging. First, some allergies can now be treated with sublingual immunotherapy rather than a shot. The FDA recently approved this therapy for allergies to five types of grass (timothy, Kentucky bluegrass, sweet vernal grass, orchard grass, and perennial ryegrass) and ragweed. Use for other allergens is likely to be approved in time. Patients place a small pill containing the allergen under the tongue every day, and the immune system gradually learns to tolerate the allergen. Second, and even more important, research has shown that for those with chronic nasal allergies, undergoing immunotherapy significantly lowers the rate of later developing asthma. In addition, those with only one primary allergy who receive allergy shots are less likely to become allergic to other major allergens later. This is true for both children and adults.

Natural and Alternative Medical Treatments

There are some effective natural nasal allergy treatments that fall outside mainstream medicine. Chapter 14 focuses on how these complementary and alternative therapies apply to all allergic disorders. Treatments that may specifically help with nasal allergies include homeopathic sprays and herbs like stinging nettle and quercetin. Locally produced raw honey is also thought to be of benefit.

OCULAR ALLERGIES

Although less common, eye allergies are just as annoying as nasal allergies. Redness and itching in both eyes are the most prominent symptoms, and some clear or white discharge may be present. Pollens, plants, animals, and dust are the most common causes, and food allergies may be involved as well. Makeup, soap, shampoo, and other facial products can irritate the eyes, as can various odors, such as perfumes, cleaning supplies, and secondhand smoke. Consider these causes if you suffer from chronic eye symptoms.

Those with chronic eczema (skin allergies) often have eye involvement as well, both within the eye and on the eyelids and skin surrounding the eyes. See Chapter 5 for more information on eczema.

Here are some specific eye-drop treatments that can bring relief:

Antihistamine and mast-cell-stabilizing eye drops. Most of these are prescription, and your doctor will decide which may be the best choice. There are two over-the-counter preparations that you can also try: Naphcon A and Zaditor.

Steroid eye drops. These prescription drops may be needed for short periods.

Homeopathic eye drops. Numerous options exist for natural relief of eye allergies. These are very safe and will be effective in many people. I have personally found these effective in my practice and in my family for most cases of eye redness, irritation, and drainage from allergies and conjunctivitis.

Saline eye drops. Simply flushing out eye allergens with saline can bring some relief. You can make your own "tear" solution by mixing a quarter teaspoon of salt in eight ounces of water.

Cool washcloths. Applying a cool, wet washcloth over the eyes provides some immediate relief.

BE SURE TO GIVE YOUR CHILD A NUTRITIONAL
ALLERGY TUNE-UP

Nutrition greatly impacts allergic disorders — and that can be for better or for worse, depending on what you eat. In Chapter 14, we present our nutritional guidelines, which, if followed, can reduce allergies and inflammation in most people. These general changes, along with the avoidance of any diagnosed food allergens, can help improve chronic nasal allergies.

4

Asthma

As you know by now, I have nasal allergies. But I also have asthma. And it sucks. My asthma began when I was twelve and we moved to sunny Southern California. Before that, my lungs were perfectly healthy. Those of you who live here as well are familiar with the smog. We just happened to move to one of the smoggiest parts of "paradise": Pasadena. My dad knew it was a mistake when we couldn't see the mountains through the orange-brown haze one summer morning. My asthma was mainly exercise-induced, and my inhaler became my best friend for those years of soccer and football. But ultimately, I managed; it didn't really hold me back.

Over the years, I continued to require an inhaler before and after any form of exercise, whether it was surfing, running on the treadmill, mountain biking, or swimming. I would also have mild asthma attacks when I ate too much. As mentioned previously, allergy testing revealed I was strongly allergic to dust and moderately allergic to mold, with a few pollens thrown in just to be annoying. Eliminating dust from my life helped relieve my nasal allergies, but the mild asthma persisted. Sometimes I'd need my inhaler twice a day for weeks on end. I even required some inhaled steroids here and there.

Three years ago I saw a clip from *The Dr. Oz Show* about a Himalayan crystal salt inhaler used as a treatment for asthma. If it was good enough for Dr. Oz, I figured I'd try it. I was pleasantly surprised: ten minutes of breathing the salts every day reduced my inhaler use significantly. It wasn't a cure, but it helped. More on this later.

My breakthrough finally came about two and a half years ago when I decided to go "paleo." The paleo diet is one of several low-carb diets that improve immune health. You'll read more about it in Chapter 14. It really changed my life, and my need for an inhaler decreased even more. I could often exercise without it. The icing on the cake came about six months later when my family and I went gluten-free. I'd never suspected I was sensitive to gluten; skin and blood allergy tests had always been normal. But ever since going gluten-free, I can go much longer than ever before without my medicated inhaler. I no longer have to take it with me everywhere. The crystal salt inhaler relieves any mild chest tightness that I occasionally feel, and I can exercise quite vigorously without any wheezing at all. I need my regular inhaler about twice a month, and I've had a bad week about twice each year. I don't consider myself cured, and I have to maintain a healthy diet and lifestyle to keep the allergic side of my immune system in check. But I'm thrilled that I don't require any chronic medications to keep my lungs healthy.

As pediatricians, Dr. Bill and I have about fifty years of combined experience in treating asthma. For most of those years, this treatment has primarily focused on allergy testing to identify possible allergens and the managing of inhalers to maintain quality of life for our patients. This is how virtually all doctors treat asthma. But times have changed; nutritional research has provided many new tools that families can use to improve their immune systems and reduce allergic inflammation, and many complementary/alternative natural treatments are now available as well. This chapter provides you with the skills you need to minimize your family's asthma.

WHY DO PEOPLE DEVELOP ASTHMA?

When children are diagnosed with asthma, this is the first question parents ask. Why did it develop? Could you have done anything to prevent it? And, of course, what can you do now to treat it and find resolution? Approximately 9 percent of Americans suffer from asthma, which is largely genetically mediated. And these genes keep spreading around to create more asthma sufferers. If one parent has asthma, a child is more likely to have asthma as well. Children who develop eczema, food allergies, or inhalant allergies are more likely to eventually develop asthma. As these allergic tendencies are mostly a result of our genes, one could argue that there's nothing you, as a parent, can do to prevent it in your children.

But let's not forget about the environment. The behavior of our genes isn't set in stone; our genetic expression is largely determined by the environment around us (a phenomenon called *epigenetics*—see page 16). The food we eat, the air we breathe, the medications we take, the activities we engage in, the chemicals we are exposed to, the stress we endure (or don't endure), even our state of mind—all of it influences how our genes behave. For example, two people may share the same genetic risks for asthma. The one who grows up in the mountains, eating all-natural foods, breathing clean air, living stress-free, and getting plenty of exercise, may never see their asthma genes turned on. The other person, who grows up around cigarette smoke and air pollution, eating the standard American diet and working at a stressful job, might have their asthma genes activated by these factors. Yet gene-environment interaction isn't always so clear; it's possible that a person with asthma genes could live in an environment with all of the risk factors and never experience wheezing.

We know that asthma occurs in 9 percent of Americans because of genetic and environmental reasons. We don't yet know enough about how to control gene-environment interactions in any practical way that allows us to completely prevent asthma in those who are genetically predisposed. But we do know that environment is important, and in this chapter you will learn how to limit environmental impact on your and your child's asthma.

A CLOSER LOOK AT THE ALLERGIC IMMUNE SYSTEM IN THE LUNGS

The allergic immune response that occurs within the lungs is similar to that which is described for the nasal passages on page 29: inhaled allergens trigger an allergic cascade of events that result in a swelling of the airway and increased mucus production. As the interior surface of the airways swells, the available room for air to pass through decreases. However, three additional factors work against those of us with asthma, adding to the strain. First, the airways are surrounded by bands of muscle, and unfortunately, the allergic response sends a message to these muscles to tighten up, which squeezes the airways and leaves even less room for air to move. The second factor is that the lung tissue of those with asthma has a much higher number of allergic white blood cells (mast cells, eosinophils, T lymphocytes, and others) compared to those without asthma. This makes the lungs hyperresponsive to almost any irritant. These cells, which were designed to help us, release their inflammatory chemicals at the slightest provocation, creating an almost constant state of inflammation within the lining of the airways. A final step that occurs in some people with decades of undertreated asthma is the deposition of collagen fibers in the lining of the lungs, a process called remodeling. This collagen decreases the airways' ability to expand and can result in permanently reduced lung function later in life.

As I said earlier, asthma sucks. But let's stop moping and get down to the business of fixing it.

DIFFERENT TYPES OF ASTHMA

Asthma varies greatly in symptoms, age of onset, causes, and severity. Understanding the different types of asthma is the first step in determining whether or not your child has asthma and, more importantly, what you can do about it.

Reactive Airway Disease

This condition, called RAD for short, refers to airways that have an asthma-like reaction to a respiratory infection. Cold viruses, particularly one called respiratory syncytial virus (RSV), cause an inflammatory reaction within the lungs that results in wheezing. Infants are the most susceptible to this type of reaction. Subsequent cold viruses will trigger wheezing and chest tightness that may require inhaler treatment for several days; a tight cough may persist for weeks after the cold is gone. My third child caught RSV at six weeks of age and has had mild RAD episodes numerous times throughout childhood. Now twelve years old, he seems to have outgrown it. RAD will resolve during the elementary years for most children, but some will go on to develop chronic asthma.

Infants with RAD don't have chronic wheezing and usually

don't have allergies. They have wheezing symptoms only during a cold or other respiratory illness, and they should be able to tolerate vigorous exercise without any difficulty (except during an illness).

Exercise-Induced Asthma

This type of asthma occurs in response to exercise. The physiologic stress of increased heart rate and blood flow to the lungs, combined with increased respiration, causes an inflammatory reaction that results in wheezing. This type of asthma often overlaps with other types; children with RAD may have exercise-induced symptoms during and after an illness, and those with chronic allergic asthma often cannot tolerate vigorous exercise. Yet some people will have symptoms only during exercise and may be able to tolerate certain exercises over others. For example, I can participate in most recreational activities and sports without difficulty, but sprinting triggers significant wheezing that requires inhaler treatment.

Episodic Allergic Asthma

Those who are allergic to only one or two allergens may have episodes of wheezing in response to exposure. For example, a child who develops an allergy to cats will suffer allergic symptoms and wheezing when exposed, but should otherwise be symptom-free as long as she is not living with cats. Such episodes of wheezing are not considered true asthma, and as long as the offending allergen is identified and avoided, this should never progress into asthma. If, on the other hand, the child continues to live with cats and suffers years of symptoms, or develops numerous other allergies, chronic asthma will set in and may become a lifelong problem.

Chronic Allergic Asthma

Those who have persistent wheezing that is not limited to simple RAD episodes or exercise-induced symptoms have chronic asthma. Chronic asthma usually has an underlying allergic cause. Daily exposure to allergens such as dust, mold, pets, food, and pollen triggers daily symptoms of asthma, with occasional asthma attacks that require urgent medical treatment. Such sufferers may have symptom-free weeks from time to time as allergen exposure varies.

In addition to the allergic triggers, a second component of chronic asthma is the underlying inflammation in the lungs. Even in the absence of allergens, the immune system within the lining of the airways can create a constant state of irritation that causes persistent symptoms and keeps the lungs primed to react when allergens do come along. Chronic allergic asthma with underlying persistent inflammation is the most serious form of asthma and results in lifelong lung disease if not properly treated.

I have—or rather, I used to have—chronic allergic asthma. I had mild, almost daily wheezing due to dust and mold allergy and underlying inflammation, with seasonal flare-ups from certain pollens interspersed with weeks or months in which I was symptom-free. Now that I've properly identified my allergens and have taken a more aggressive approach to reducing inflammation, I enjoy months of symptom-free time.

PHYSICAL SIGNS AND SYMPTOMS OF ASTHMA

Asthma signs are obvious to most keen observers, as audible wheezing and labored breathing are a clear giveaway. But sometimes the symptoms aren't so apparent. Here are the signs you should look for.

Wheezing

Wheezing is a high-pitched whistling sound most commonly heard during exhalation (while a person is breathing out). It is caused by turbulent air flowing through the narrowed airway, similar to the effect of water flowing through a kinked hose. When mild, it might be heard only at the very end of the exhalation. During more severe attacks, wheezing will be audible during inhalation as well. It is important to distinguish true wheezing from other types of respiratory sounds, because the required treatment varies widely depending on whether or not a person is truly wheezing. Here are some common symptoms that are *not* wheezing and are not related to asthma:

Chest congestion. Rattling sounds in the chest that temporarily clear with coughing are probably due to mucus in the upper lungs. Wheezing, on the other hand, does not clear with coughing. If your child's chest rattling comes and goes throughout the day, it is likely simple mucus congestion. You may be able to feel the mucus vibrating with each breath when you place your hand on your child's chest. A person with asthma and wheezing will be able to cough up some mucus, but the underlying wheezing sounds will persist.

Stridor. This medical term refers to the unusual breathing sound that occurs during laryngitis or croup; the vocal cords at the very top of the airway are narrowed, creating a loud, hoarse, raspy sound with inhalation and exhalation that can be heard from across the room. The child may sound as if he has lost his voice, and the cough may mimic a seal barking. Wheezing, in contrast, occurs because of narrowing down within the lungs, is fairly quiet, and does not create any changes in the voice.

Tight, Purposeful Cough

Asthma attacks usually limit the amount of air a child can take in, so the resulting cough will likely be shallow and weak, and you can hear the wheezing sound as air is quickly forced out of the lungs. In addition, the asthmatic cough is usually purposeful; a person will take a deep breath, then force out a single cough. Regular coughs, on the other hand, are usually deeper, are uncontrollable, and come in waves or fits. The purposeful asthmatic cough is a survival mechanism. When the forced air hits the narrowed airways on its way out, some air is actually pushed back down into the lungs to allow more oxygen absorption. One subtype of asthma is called cough-variant asthma, in which a person may not wheeze at all; persistent cough is the primary symptom of this subtype.

Retractions

Retractions are a classic hallmark of an asthma attack, and they underscore the importance of removing a child's shirt and visually observing the chest. Retractions refer to the sucking in of the chest wall during an asthmatic inhalation. When a healthy person inhales, the chest is supposed to expand. But when a person with asthma takes a breath, the chest tries to expand faster than the restricted air can enter the lungs, creating negative pressure that pulls (or retracts) the skin inward. You can actually see the skin around your child's neck, between the ribs, and in the upper abdomen suck inward with each breath. When the asthma is severe, you may even see the lower half of your child's rib cage collapse inward with each attempted breath.

Cough with Exertion

Asthma symptoms will invariably worsen with exertion. Tight coughing fits are particularly troublesome during active play. Even the exertion of vigorous laughing can trigger an asthma attack.

Labored Shoulder Breathing

A person with asthma may use the shoulders to assist in breathing. You will see the shoulders move or shrug upward with each breath. This is known as using accessory muscles to help with breathing (use this phrase if you want to sound particularly knowledgeable to your doctor).

Prolonged Exhalation

The ultraobservant parent will notice that it takes her asthmatic child longer to breathe out than to breathe in. As stated previously, wheezing occurs more during exhalation, so it takes longer for the air to leave the narrowed airways of the lungs than it does for air to enter during inhalation.

Rapid Breathing

During an asthma flare, a person will breathe more rapidly to compensate for the lack of oxygen with each breath. You should get to know your child's regular rate of breathing when he is healthy so you can accurately assess the rate when he is sick.

Signs of a Severe Asthma Attack

If your child has blue lips, is extremely drowsy, or cannot get enough air to speak or cry, along with many of the above signs, this indicates a potentially life-threatening situation that warrants immediate emergency care.

---

i-MEDICINE

Before you head to the doctor's office, video your child's breathing with an iPhone or other mobile device. Remove your child's shirt and make sure the lighting is adequate so your doctor can see the breathing as well as hear it. If your child has improved by the time your doctor sees you, you'll have some video evidence for her to examine.

MAKING THE DIAGNOSIS OF ASTHMA

An asthma diagnosis requires teamwork between your family and your doctor. No one is diagnosed with asthma after just one episode of wheezing; a period of observation is necessary to assess the frequency and severity of symptoms and the response to initial treatment. Here is our play-by-play guide to making the diagnosis.

Keep a Diary of Symptoms

Note in a journal the specific symptoms you see in yourself or your child and any physical signs you notice. Note the frequency: Do symptoms occur daily, weekly, or less often? Do symptoms fit into a specific type of asthma as described on page 53? Do symptoms occur only during and after a respiratory illness or only with exertion? Does your child have symptoms year-round, or are the symptoms restricted to certain seasons? If your child is old enough, elicit a description of how her breathing feels. Does her chest feel tight? Does she feel as if she's getting enough air? Write down your observations and bring your notes to the doctor.

Consider the Severity of Symptoms

Determine to what extent the symptoms interfere with quality of life. Does a nighttime cough cause waking several times each night? Does your child have difficulty falling asleep due to shortness of breath? Does he or she have to rest more often than other kids during sports activities?

Examine Your Child's and Family's Allergic History

If asthma is a problem for either parent, or if a child already has other allergic problems such as eczema or nasal allergies, you should take any suspicious and persistent symptoms more seriously.

At the Doctor's Office

A thorough medical examination and discussion with your pediatrician or family doctor is important. In addition to your notes and observations, here is what your doctor may do:

Physical exam. Your doctor should observe your child's breathing for signs described above. Careful listening with a stethoscope will uncover any wheezing, tight inspiration, and prolonged exhalation time.

Response to inhaler treatment. Your doctor will likely administer an inhaled treatment with a fast-acting medication in the office and observe the response (see "Treating Various Types and Degrees of Asthma," on page 71). Resolution of symptoms confirms that an asthmatic situation is occurring. Alternatively, your doctor may send you home with inhaled treatment and gauge the response over several days.

Peak flow measurement. A peak flow meter is a plastic tube your doctor can use to measure the force of exhalation. As you read on page 56, the outflow of air during exhalation is restricted during an asthma flare-up. This meter can measure that level of restriction and provide a clue to diagnosis. You can also use this inexpensive tool at home to assess the severity of wheezing (see Asthma Action Plan, page 76).

Recurrent episodes. Asthma is rarely diagnosed during the first attack. The doctor will treat the acute episode and will then observe for subsequent problems during the weeks and months that follow.

Chest X-ray. A chest X-ray is usually reserved for severe asthma attacks that don't respond to immediate inhalation therapy or for cases when pneumonia is suspected (symptoms may include a fever and labored breathing without wheezing). An X-ray will reveal some signs that are specific to asthma, which can help a doctor distinguish between an asthma attack and other urgent respiratory conditions. We rarely use X-rays in our evaluations.

Determining the type of asthma. If recurrent episodes are related to cold and cough illnesses, your doctor will likely diagnose you or your child with RAD (see page 53). If persistent symptoms have flared up unrelated to an illness, episodic allergic asthma may be the diagnosis. When this persists throughout the year, a diagnosis of chronic allergic asthma is made. Those who seem to have symptoms only during exercise may be diagnosed with exercise-induced asthma. A person may also have a mixed presentation, with features of some or all of these patterns. For example, a person with chronic allergic asthma will likely have exercise-induced asthma as well.

At an Asthma Specialist's Office

While most cases of asthma can be managed by a primary care doctor, an allergist or a pulmonologist can provide a higher level of diagnostic measures and medical management than most pediatricians and family doctors. Here is what a specialist may offer:

Pulmonary function testing. A computerized device can be used to assess lung volume and degree of obstruction and is considerably more accurate than the simple peak flow meter described above. But it is rarely needed, as a careful history and physical examination are usually sufficient. Pulmonary function testing can be a useful tool when the diagnosis is in doubt or when the severity of persistent asthma needs to be assessed.

Allergy skin testing. When allergies are suspected of playing a role in asthma, an allergist can be a valuable partner in assessing allergic triggers for asthma (see Chapter 2, Allergy Testing).

Complex medical treatment. Children with moderate to severe asthma that persists despite initial therapy from a primary care doctor should be managed by a specialist. More intensive prescription therapy may be necessary to get the asthma under control, and a specialist has more knowledge and experience in this area.

UNDERSTANDING ASTHMA MEDICATIONS

Before we discuss asthma treatment and prevention in detail, you should be aware of what medications are available, how they work, and what the side effects are. This way, you can better understand the treatment steps we discuss in the following section, and you can also have a more informed discussion with your doctor. While chronic medication isn't a necessary solution for everybody with asthma, short-term use will be needed from time to time in virtually all asthma sufferers. Here is a complete presentation of all available asthma medications. At the time of this writing, all are prescription only.

Short-Acting Beta2-Agonists (SABAs)

This long and complicated name refers to the basic inhaler that most people with asthma use for quick relief. These medications work by activating what are called the beta2 receptors on the surface of the cells in the lungs. Activation of these receptors results in relaxation of the bands of muscle that surround the airways, allowing the airways to expand. It also causes mucus to move higher into the upper chest, where it can be better coughed out. And it is theorized that these meds decrease the mast cell release of histamines, but that is uncertain. There are three SABAs currently on the market:

Albuterol. This is the oldest and most commonly used medication for asthma. It is available as an inhaler, as a solution for a nebulizer machine (see box on page 68), and as a liquid that is swallowed. The oral liquid is rarely used anymore, as the side effects (see below) are fairly common and uncomfortable. The inhaled medication absorbs through the lining of the airways, enters the muscle fibers that surround the airways, and causes those fibers to relax. This expands the airway and allows the person to breathe more deeply and easily. It begins to work right away and lasts about four hours. This is what I use when I need some quick relief during exercise, a respiratory illness, or a flare-up of my allergies and asthma. Brand names include Pro-Air, Proventil, and Ventolin.

Levalbuterol. This is a newer, more potent (and more expensive) form of albuterol. It has two advantages: it is effective in smaller doses, and it causes fewer and less noticeable side effects. However, newer isn't necessarily better. Albuterol has such a long track record of safety and efficacy that it remains the standard treatment for most people, including me. Levalbuterol is reserved for those who can't tolerate albuterol, or for the few in whom albuterol doesn't work adequately. It is available in both inhaler and nebulizer formulations. Xopenex is currently the only name brand.

Pirbuterol. This medication is virtually identical to albuterol, but it is not currently approved for children. The only name brand that was made was MaxAir Autohaler. This, however, recently became unavailable due to new regulations on how inhalers are manufactured (see page 88). It should become available again in the coming years.

Side effects of SABAs. Most children and adults do not experience any side effects at all. Infants are more likely to show side effects, but these are usually mild and manageable. Effects are basically what one would expect from drinking too much caffeine: increased heart rate and jitteriness. SABAs may make a younger child hyperactive for a few hours, and infants may be irritable and jittery. For those in whom the effects are intolerable, a switch to levalbuterol should solve the problem. But in our experience, these effects are rarely noticed, and the benefit of breathing more easily is well worth the small risk of side effects.

HOW TO PROPERLY USE A SPRAY INHALER

Many people make the mistake of placing all inhalers inside the mouth and wrapping the lips around the mouthpiece. This is only proper for powdered inhalers, which must be breathed in with the mouth enclosed around the mouthpiece. Inhalers that spray, on the other hand, should not be placed in the mouth. Most of the medication ends up sticking to the moist surface of the mouth before it can be inhaled. Instead, here is the proper way to use an inhaler:

- Shake the inhaler.
- Hold the inhaler approximately two inches away from the mouth, pointing toward the mouth.
- Take several slow, deep breaths to prepare.
- Exhale completely (but without forcing every last bit of air out of the lungs), then start to take a deep breath.
- Spray the inhaler a split second *after* the inhalation begins. The idea is to have air already flowing into the mouth when the inhaler is activated; this allows more medication to be taken down into the lungs, instead of depositing in and around the mouth. But don't spray too late or the medicine won't go down deep enough.
- Inhale completely at a moderate speed, drawing the medication down into the lungs.
- Hold the breath for at least five seconds, but no more than ten seconds. Holding the breath too long stresses the lungs and can exacerbate wheezing. Then resume normal breathing.
- Repeat with a second inhalation (if two inhalations are prescribed, which is usually the case) after waiting a minute or two.
- Rinse the mouth out if using a steroid inhaler.

Read the inhaler directions to determine whether you should regularly rinse the inhaler with warm water. Some inhalers will have medication buildup at the tip, which blocks subsequent sprays.

Long-Acting Beta2-Agonists (LABAs)

As the name implies, these meds work in the same manner as SABAs, but they last longer—up to twelve hours. They don't work as quickly, so they are not recommended for relief of acute wheezing. Instead, they are considered a preventive therapy for those with moderate to severe asthma with persistent symptoms. They are rarely used alone, as some research has demonstrated that they may actually *increase* the risk of a sudden and severe asthma attack when routinely used alone. Their efficacy may also wane over time if used alone. Therefore, these inhaled medications are used in conjunction with inhaled steroids for those who require aggressive therapy. **Salmeterol** (brand names Advair and Serevent) and **formoterol** (brand names Brovana, Dulera, Foradil, and Symbicort) are the forms of LABAs that are currently available. These are approved for children four years of age and older.

Side effects of LABAs. Side effects are similar to those seen with SABAs, and they tend to be uncommon.

Inhaled Corticosteroids (ICSs)

The word *steroids* generally turns off most parents. As pediatricians who prefer to take a more natural approach in our practice, we have some reservations about long-term use of steroid therapy in children. However, steroids definitely have their place in asthma therapy, and we do prescribe them for children with moderate to severe asthma. But if you or your child requires this level of chronic therapy, it means you may not be making enough lifestyle, household, and nutritional changes to reduce allergies and inflammation. We focus on these environmental areas with our patients, then wean them off the steroids as soon as possible.

This is where our Pills and Skills model of health care really shines. Use some pills (or inhalers) to get asthma under control, then use your skills for better long-term resolution.

Steroids work by diminishing the immune system's allergic response; specifically, they reduce the number of allergic white blood cells and cytokines (see page 8) in the lung tissues. This means that as allergens enter the lungs, the allergic response is minimized and wheezing can be prevented. Because inhaled steroids do not act quickly, they are not used for relief of acute symptoms. They are available as inhalers and nebulizer solutions for chronic, daily use to help prevent asthma, and as oral liquids and pills for short-term use to relieve a severe asthma attack. There are too many steroid brands to list here, and we don't have any particular preferences among them.

Side effects. Noticeable side effects are uncommon, and ICSs are usually very well tolerated. Oral thrush (yeast overgrowth in the mouth) can occur and is preventable by rinsing the mouth after each use and by using a spacer device (see page 68). Chronic and more serious effects that may occur within the body are dose-dependent; they are extremely rare with low-dose ICSs and are more likely with high-dose, long-term use of ICSs. These include cataracts or glaucoma, reduced bone density, and slowed growth during the first year of use, especially in girls. A child who experiences slow growth during the first year of therapy should begin to grow at a normal speed again, even with ongoing therapy, but she may not regain that lost half inch to one inch. However, chronic, uncontrolled asthma can also affect growth — so if ICSs are needed, they are probably the lesser of two evils, particularly at lower doses.

METHODS OF ADMINISTERING INHALED MEDICATIONS

There are three ways to administer inhaled medications, and your doctor will advise you on which is best for you or your child:

Inhaler alone. This is the standard method used for older children and adults. The advantage is that the inhaler fits into any pocket or purse, so it is readily available anytime, anywhere. When used properly (see box on page 65), a simple inhaler can deliver a full dose of medication effectively. The primary disadvantage is that some medication will stick inside the mouth. For SABAs and LABAs, this doesn't matter, as enough medication reaches the lungs if the inhalation is coordinated properly. However, steroids can irritate the mouth and cause yeast overgrowth. Rinsing the mouth after steroid inhaler use can help.

Inhaler with spacer device. A spacer is a tube with a mouthpiece on one end. An inhaler is sprayed into an opening on the opposite end; then the person takes about six slow, deep breaths through the mouthpiece, drawing the medication down into the lungs. This allows medication to be delivered without needing to properly coordinate the timing of inhalation. The two disadvantages are that it is less portable than an inhaler alone, and it costs more money (many insurance plans don't pay for spacer devices). But a spacer can effectively administer inhaler medication to infants and young children without resorting to a nebulizer machine. For those on ICS therapy, this device limits the amount of steroids that stick to the mouth.

Nebulizer machine. This machine is used to deliver inhaled medication gradually over several minutes and requires electricity. Liquid medication is placed in a small chamber, and the machine vaporizes it and releases it slowly as a mist. The person inhales this mist through a mouthpiece at the end of a long tube. Nebulizers are available with a prescription and are covered by insurance. Studies have shown that children who use a spacer

device inhale medication just as effectively as those who use a
nebulizer, so nebulizers are primarily reserved for infants and
young children who won't cooperate with a spacer device. These
devices are also standard in any emergency room or doctor's
office to help relieve urgent asthma attacks.

Leukotriene Inhibitors

These oral medications are a newer addition to asthma therapy.
They work by blocking the effects of leukotrienes, the chemicals
similar to histamines that are released as part of the allergic
response (see page 8). Blocking these leukotrienes can relax the
muscles surrounding the airways and reduce mucus secretion,
thus alleviating asthma symptoms. Leukotriene inhibitors do not
act quickly, so they are not used for fast relief (SABA inhalers are
best for that). They can be used alone or in combination with
other medications to reduce chronic and persistent asthma symptoms. They may be tried as an alternative to ICSs for mild, persistent asthma, especially in young children who won't cooperate
with inhalation therapies and may better tolerate a decent-tasting
daily oral medication. These medications may also be effective
enough to prevent exercise-induced asthma symptoms. In addition, they are helpful for nasal allergies (page 43).

Montelukast (brand name Singulair) and **zafirlukast** (brand
name Accolate) are the two most commonly used leukotriene
inhibitors in children and adults. **Zileuton** (brand name Zyflo) is
a third choice, used only in teens and adults at this time.

Side effects. Leukotriene inhibitors are very well tolerated and
usually have no noticeable side effects. In rare cases, long-term
use of zafirlukast and zileuton can cause liver damage.

Other, Less Commonly Used Medications

SABAs, LABAs, ICSs, and leukotriene inhibitors are the primary medications used in asthma. The following medications are seldom used but deserve a brief mention:

Ipratropium. This inhaled medication can be used in conjunction with SABAs in an emergency room to stop an asthma attack. It works by blocking the nerves that constrict the muscles surrounding the airways in the lungs.

Theophylline and aminophylline. Also generally reserved for an ER or hospital setting, these meds are similar to caffeine. They dilate the airways by relaxing the surrounding muscles.

Cromolyn. This mast cell stabilizing medication (see page 42) can be used as an inhaler to reduce asthma symptoms. It is rarely used anymore, as other inhalers are more effective. It can be used to prevent exercise-induced asthma instead of a SABA. Nedocromil is a similar inhaled medication that can be used in older children and adults.

Omalizumab. This is a recently developed immune therapy (brand name Xolair) that is reserved for teens and adults with severe allergic asthma. It is an injection that is administered by an allergy specialist every two to four weeks. This unique therapy is not a medication. It is a manufactured antibody that binds to, and inactivates, a person's own IgE antibodies, thus preventing the allergic cascade within the lungs and other body tissues. Recent reports of severe, life-threatening anaphylactic shock after receiving this treatment have prompted the FDA to issue a warning to doctors and patients about long-term use. This severe reaction may occur at any time, even days after an injection or after many previously tolerated injections. Doctors should consider discontinuing therapy after asthma is well controlled for a time.

Antibiotics. A particular class of antibiotics, called macrolides (erythromycin, azithromycin, clarithromycin), has the added benefit of reducing inflammation. In addition, some asthmatics are chronically infected with bacteria in the lungs, and these bacteria are sensitive to the antibiotics. A course of the antibiotics may reduce the severity of an asthma flare-up.

TREATING VARIOUS TYPES AND DEGREES OF ASTHMA

Now that you've been introduced to the pharmacopeia of asthma medications, let's move on to treatment. There are two primary components of treating asthma. The first is to relieve acute symptoms when they occur. This step is relatively simple, and your child will appreciate the relief you can offer when wheezing rears its ugly head. The second step is to reduce underlying inflammation and allergic reactivity within the lungs, which takes a great deal of time and commitment but is well worth the effort.

Reactive Airway Disease

If your child experiences asthma symptoms triggered by a cold or flu virus, you will need to provide relief measures to keep his breathing stable and comfortable for the duration of the illness. If you are currently experiencing your child's very first episode of RAD, we recommend you see your doctor today. Subsequent episodes can generally be managed at home, with guidance from your health care provider.

Inhaled albuterol. Your doctor will likely prescribe *albuterol* (see page 63) to expand the constricted airways and relieve the wheezing. This nonsteroid treatment can be administered with a simple inhaler for children old enough to cooperate (see the box titled "Methods of Administering Inhaled Medications," page 68), or via a nebulizer machine that turns the medication into a vaporized mist that is inhaled over several minutes. If your child responds well, you will continue this treatment at home as needed for the duration of the illness. Some kids will need an inhalation every four hours; others can get by with a dose only once or twice a day. As the cold and cough illness resolves, the frequency of inhaled treatments should decrease until your child is symptom-free. This may take only a few days, but it can require a few weeks of inhaled support in some cases.

Alternatively, your doctor may prescribe *levalbuterol* (current brand name Xopenex). This newer version of albuterol can work just as well, but with fewer side effects (see page 64). We rarely prescribe it, however, as virtually all children handle albuterol without side effects and the extra cost isn't warranted. Most doctors reserve levalbuterol for those in whom albuterol side effects occur.

Chest-clearing measures. Steam yourself or your child in a bathroom with a hot shower running several times each day, or use a facial steamer if possible. Run a hot steam vaporizer at night. Administer over-the-counter expectorant medication (currently approved for kids four years of age and older) to make the cough more productive; natural expectorants (available in natural health stores and online) can also be used, especially in younger kids. Keeping the chest clear of mucus helps the illness and RAD resolve more quickly.

Hypertonic saline inhalation. A new technique for nebulized inhalation of SABAs involves mixing the med in a stronger salt solution (called hypertonic saline) instead of regular saline.

Research on this practice reveals that it hastens the resolution of the wheezing and shortens the hospital stay, particularly in infants and young children. It isn't standard practice yet, but if ongoing research continues to demonstrate positive results, it likely will become the norm.

Steroid treatment. Rarely, a child's RAD episodes are severe enough to warrant a fast-acting oral steroid treatment (see page 76) to reduce lung inflammation. This is typically reserved for those in whom symptoms are moderate to severe and for whom an albuterol or levalbuterol treatment doesn't provide relief.

Recurrent episodes of RAD. Be ready to start albuterol inhaler treatments with subsequent cold and cough illnesses. Under your doctor's guidance, you may start treatments at the first sign of a cold without waiting for asthmatic symptoms to begin, as this may prevent the development of severe and urgent symptoms. Inhaled steroids may also be started with the onset of RAD in children who are known to experience moderate to severe prolonged courses of asthma whenever a respiratory infection hits. When started at the beginning of an RAD flare-up, inhaled steroids can reduce the duration and severity of the attack and the reliance on albuterol. Most parents are reluctant to give their children steroids, but we believe a short course of steroids is a safe and important tool to use when needed.

Long-term prevention and resolution of RAD. Because RAD often doesn't have an allergic component, allergy-prevention measures generally don't help. Children will likely have RAD with each cold or cough illness until three to five years of age, at which time many kids outgrow their RAD tendency and move on to have a healthy, asthma-free life. My youngest child is now twelve years old, and most of his cold and cough illnesses don't trigger wheezing or tight cough anymore. He still has an occasional RAD episode every year or two and needs one or two puffs of the inhaler. Fortunately, he has no chronic or exercise-induced symptoms.

But some children will develop chronic asthma, especially if other allergic disorders, like nasal allergies or eczema, come into play. By following our natural and nutritional steps to reduce chronic inflammation, calm down the allergic branch of the immune system, and boost the germ-fighting properties of the immune system described in Chapter 14, you may be able to decrease the number and severity of cold and cough illnesses and reduce the RAD episodes.

Exercise-Induced Asthma

If you and your doctor decide that your asthma is limited to exercise, and it does not have a preventable allergic component, inhaler medication will be the mainstay of therapy.

Albuterol inhaler. Two puffs of this SABA inhaler fifteen to thirty minutes before exercise can prevent wheezing and tightness in the chest and will improve exercise tolerance. Doses can be repeated during or after exercise as needed. Levalbuterol can be used for those who don't tolerate albuterol.

Cromolyn inhaler. This prescription is an alternative to albuterol (see page 42); used before exercise, it may prevent wheezing. It works by reducing the release of histamine and other wheeze-inducing chemicals from the immune cells in the lining of the lungs. However, it is generally believed to be less effective than albuterol. Your doctor will help you decide which to use. Cromolyn is not fast-acting, so it won't bring rapid relief when used *during* exercise.

Leukotriene inhibitor. This oral medication may work well for some with exercise-induced asthma. See page 44.

Long-term resolution of exercise-induced asthma. For those whose asthma is triggered only by exercise, the most important treatment for long-term resolution involves following our natural and nutritional approach to reduce inflammation (as described in Chapter 14). This has made a considerable difference for me, and it has done wonders for many of our patients. You should also consult with your doctor to make sure your symptoms are caused by asthma and not by a cardiac problem or another type of lung disease. That distinction is beyond the scope of this book.

Acute Treatment for Allergic Asthma

Once a diagnosis of allergic asthma has been made, it's time to use fast-acting inhaled medications to bring some initial relief. Simultaneously, you will begin to address long-term solutions to achieve resolution of the asthma (discussed in the section that follows).

Inhaled SABAs. Albuterol (or levalbuterol, see page 63) is the mainstay of fast-acting relief for any asthma attack. If you are reading this book, you have probably already seen a doctor and have a SABA inhaler or solution for a nebulizer machine. You will use this medication every four hours until the asthma attack is under control, then space out the frequency of doses as tolerated until wheezing is resolved. This may take a day, or it may take several.

Antihistamines. Administer oral antihistamines (see page 41) to reduce the body's internal allergic reaction to whatever allergen has caused the attack.

Oral steroids. A three-to-five-day course of oral steroids is the most potent way to reduce lung inflammation and allergic reaction during a severe attack. These take several hours to begin to work, and they peak after about twelve hours. Oral steroids are generally reserved for those who don't respond adequately to SABA inhalation therapy. We use these short courses of steroids in our office without concern for any long-term side effects.

You should develop a written Asthma Action Plan with your doctor and be prepared with prescription medications at home so you can act appropriately when an asthma attack occurs. See the following box for more information about Asthma Action Plans.

ASTHMA ACTION PLAN

This plan is a written set of instructions filled out by your doctor that provides guidance on what to do in the event of an asthma attack. Your doctor will likely give you some verbal instructions at your appointment, but it's not easy for a parent to remember those steps during the stress of an asthma attack. A written plan is the standard of care and will look something like this:

Green Zone. This means that all is well and there are no symptoms of asthma. Any daily preventive medications will be written in this section to remind you to stay on your medication, including an inhaler for exercise (if needed). If a peak flow meter is being used (see page 61), your normal value will be written in here as a reminder of what your peak flow result should be when you are well.

Yellow Zone. This means you are experiencing a mild to moderate flare-up of symptoms. If you are using a peak flow meter, your measurements will be between 60 and 80 percent of your normal

MEDICAL MANAGEMENT OF CHRONIC ALLERGIC ASTHMA

Medications are an integral part of bringing chronic asthma under control. These "pills" don't take the place of the "skills" you will employ to achieve long-term resolution of the asthma discussed in the following section, but you will likely require some degree of medical treatment at first. The medical approach to managing asthma that is recommended by the specialists and policy makers of our health care system is based on three areas of classification: (1) severity of asthma before initiating chronic

---

value. A SABA inhaler or nebulizer medication will be written in here, with proper dosage and intervals between treatments. If you feel much better within about twenty minutes and return to a normal state, you will continue this extra treatment for a day and then go back to your Green Zone instructions. If you don't improve, an additional medication, such as an oral steroid or higher dose of the SABA inhaled treatments, may be written here. If you worsen, go to the Red Zone instructions. Alternatively, if you remain in the Yellow Zone for about twenty-four hours without improving or worsening, you qualify for Red Zone therapy.

Red Zone. This means you are in trouble. Wheezing is severe, peak flow is less than 60 percent of normal, and Yellow Zone treatments haven't helped. You should have a high dose of SABA inhaler therapy written here that you can administer while you call your doctor. Over the next fifteen minutes, you should improve. You will then have also reached your doctor and arranged for an appointment that day. If you don't improve over these fifteen minutes, seek emergency care at the closest emergency room (call 911 if your situation is life-threatening).

therapy, (2) stepwise approach to using medications based on this severity, and (3) assessing response to therapy and adjusting if needed. The term *stepwise* refers to the ability to periodically adjust therapy by taking a step up (more aggressive therapy) when needed and stepping down again as you are able.

Classifying the Severity of Asthma Before Treatment

Before any treatment is started, asthma severity is initially classified as either intermittent or persistent. Persistent asthma is further classified as mild, moderate, or severe. Initial classifications are based on the following criteria:

Intermittent. This term is applied to those who have occasional but recurrent asthma symptoms but who are problem-free most days in any given week. Specifically, symptoms occur on no more than two days per week, a SABA inhaler is used on no more than two days per week, the asthma does not interfere with normal daily activities, and a course of oral steroids is only needed once in a year to stop an asthma attack (or is not needed at all). For infants and children through four years of age, night waking due to asthma should not occur for the asthma to be considered intermittent, whereas older kids and adults may experience one or two night wakings each month. In addition, lung function testing (performed by an asthma specialist) is also used to classify severity, and lung function is unlikely to be impaired in intermittent asthma.

Mild persistent. Chronic asthma is considered persistent if symptoms occur on a more regular basis, if oral steroids are required more than once a year, or if mild asthma attacks lasting more than one day occur four or more times in a year. Specifically, mild persistent asthma sufferers require a SABA inhaler more than two days each week, but not daily, and experience only minor limitation of normal daily activities. Night waking due to asthma occurs once or twice each month in children through age four, or once a week in older kids and adults. Lung function, if tested, is only mildly reduced.

Moderate persistent. These sufferers will experience daily symptoms that require once-daily SABA use and will find their daily activity level somewhat limited. Infants will wake up about once a week, and older children and adults will wake up more often (but not every night). Lung function testing will show moderate impairment.

Severe persistent. Criteria for this classification include symptoms throughout every day that require several SABA treatments, and normal daily activities that are extremely limited. Night waking may occur almost every night. Severe asthmatics will likely have needed several courses of oral steroids in a year and visited an emergency room a few times. Lung function testing will document the severe impairment.

Note: SABA inhalers that are used for prevention or treatment of exercise-induced asthma are not taken into account in these criteria. In other words, a person who uses an inhaler every day for exercise but only needs it once or twice each week for spontaneous wheezing would be considered to have only intermittent asthma.

Stepwise Approach to Beginning Medications

Once the asthma severity is classified, medical treatment is started to bring the asthma under control. Therapy begins with the appropriate step level that matches the initial severity of disease. Those who improve take a step *down* in therapy. Those who worsen take a step *up*.

Step 1. Those who stay within the criteria for intermittent asthma should only require SABA inhalation therapy on an as-needed basis. They don't warrant any preventive daily medication.

Step 2. Those with mild persistent asthma are recommended to take daily low-dose inhaled corticosteroids (ICSs) to prevent symptoms and improve activities of daily living. Alternatives to this choice include a cromolyn inhaler and an oral leukotriene inhibitor. Older kids and adults may consider theophylline. Such people may take oral antihistamine allergy medications as well (see page 41).

Step 3. Moderate persistent asthma sufferers should begin medium-dose ICS therapy. Children five years of age and older and adults can instead try combination therapy with low-dose ICS plus one of the following: oral leukotriene inhibitor, LABA (long-acting beta2-agonist) inhaler, or oral theophylline.

Anyone who fits the criteria for moderate persistent asthma and requires Step 3 therapy or higher should consult with an asthma specialist and consider allergy shots, especially if they are allergic to dust mites, animal dander, or pollens.

KEEP A DAILY LOG

Doctors use two primary factors to assess asthma control: the frequency of SABA inhaler use and the extent to which symptoms interfere with daily activities. The only person who can communicate this information to your doctor is *you*. And the only way for you to accurately do so is to keep a daily log of SABA inhaler use and the degree of your symptoms. Bring this log to every doctor's appointment.

Steps 4, 5, and 6. People who suffer from severe persistent asthma will proceed to these advanced steps, which involve multiple medications, including high-dose ICSs, LABA inhalers, leukotriene inhibitors, theophylline, and/or oral steroids. These details are beyond the scope of this book and will be guided by an asthma and allergy specialist.

Assessing Asthma Control and Adjusting Medications

Patients should follow up with a doctor every month until the asthma is under control. If bothersome symptoms persist, therapy should be stepped up one level at a time. As symptoms improve, treatment steps down. Here are the definitions of asthma control:

Well controlled. This is the ultimate goal of asthma therapy. Criteria are the same as those listed on page 78 for intermittent asthma: a person should be symptom-free most days each week with no limitations in daily activities and should have experienced no more than one asthma attack that required oral steroids within the year. After three months of well-controlled asthma, the doctor may recommend one step down in therapy. For example, an older child on low-dose ICSs and a LABA inhaler (Step 3 of therapy) could discontinue the LABA inhaler.

Not well controlled. This patient will experience symptoms for several days each week, have some limitations on daily activities, and require oral steroids to calm down an asthma attack two or more times in a year, despite being on therapy. These are similar to the criteria for *mild* to moderate persistent asthma on page 78. In short, the current level of therapy isn't working and should be stepped up a notch. In addition, the doctor should make sure inhalers and oral meds are being administered properly, and further allergy-prevention steps should be initiated.

Very poorly controlled. This asthma sufferer is experiencing the severely persistent level of daily symptoms described on page 79 and requires stepped-up therapy and a course of oral steroids to bring the asthma under better control. This patient should work more closely with an allergy and asthma specialist to determine better long-term solutions.

This three-pronged approach to classifying asthma severity, initiating treatment, and assessing control and adjusting therapy is well researched and extremely effective in bringing asthma under control with medications. To start, short-acting albuterol (SABA) inhalers are safe and effective, as are oral leukotriene inhibitors and low-dose inhaled steroids (ICSs). Stepped-up therapy with LABA inhalers, higher-dose ICSs, and other advanced therapies bring more risk and side effects, but poorly controlled asthma warrants these therapies for an appropriate period. Now it's time to use your skills to avoid exposure to allergens, lower the immune system's response to unavoidable allergens, reduce lung and body inflammation, and improve your health—so that you can step down your "pills" and achieve resolution of symptoms.

ACHIEVING RESOLUTION OF CHRONIC ALLERGIC ASTHMA

After thirty years of living with asthma, I can finally say that I have my asthma under control with no use of daily medications and no limitations on my daily activities. In this section, we share everything you can do for yourself and your child to put asthma to rest.

Track Down and Eliminate Allergies

This all-important step cannot be emphasized enough. I am extremely allergic to dust, and eliminating all sources of dust in my home has made a significant difference. Review the section "Tracking Down the Cause of Nasal Allergies" on page 32, because whatever can trigger nasal allergies can also contribute to asthma. You may discover some fairly simple solutions. For example, a toddler who develops persistent asthma may be allergic to cow's milk, and a milk-free diet may be all that is needed. Perhaps it's the new family pet that has triggered the symptoms. But it often isn't so simple, and if your investigation doesn't elicit an obvious source of allergies, it's time for testing.

Allergy testing. Review the testing options in Chapter 2 and discuss with your pediatrician or family doctor whether you should try blood testing first or go straight to an allergist for skin testing. The results should guide you on what you can eliminate from your life. Consider both methods of testing if the first doesn't provide adequate relief.

Allergy elimination. Chapter 13 lays out specific measures you can take in your home and your life to reduce exposure to your allergens and reduce the risk of chronic, lifelong asthma.

Clean air. If allergy testing reveals inhalant allergies (dust, mold, pollens, or pets), using an air filter system to clean allergens out of the air is critical. But even if testing does not demonstrate such allergens, clean air is still important for asthmatics. Review the air filter options on page 253 and invest in your family's lung health. Avoid perfumes and other irritating aromas, as these can exacerbate wheezing in some people. Secondhand smoke must be eliminated from the home of any asthmatic. Air pollution should not be underestimated. The smoggy four years we spent near Los Angeles when I was a teenager were a likely contributing trigger for my asthma. Move to cleaner air if you can; live away from freeways and industrial centers where air pollution is worst.

Complementary and alternative testing for allergies. In Chapter 2 we presented alternative options for allergy testing. These are worth pursuing if mainstream testing doesn't provide answers and chronic asthma symptoms persist.

CIGARETTES AND ASTHMA DON'T MIX

It should go without saying, but it must be said anyway. If someone in the home has asthma, no one in the family should smoke. Secondhand smoke is a direct cause of asthma.

Reduce Allergic Response to Allergens

Some allergens are unavoidable. We see patients who test positive for both dust and pollens, and we label these kids as essentially being "allergic to air." No matter how careful you are, you can't avoid all potential allergens. But you may be able to make your body less reactive to them. Medications and allergy shots are effective mainstream medical treatments, and several natural and nutritional approaches to asthma prevention will help as well.

Anti-inflammatory foods. Other than allergen avoidance, this is the most important and effective way for you to reduce your allergic response to allergens. It is so critical that we devote much of the last chapter to this issue alone (Chapter 14). In short, what you eat greatly influences the allergic and inflammatory potential in your body. Many foods in the standard American diet (dubbed the SAD diet) cause inflammation, such as the unhealthy fats and oils in fast food and most commercially processed beef. But good nutrition is more about what you *do* eat than what you *don't*. Fill your diet with anti-inflammatory foods, such as various spices, healthy fish, free-range grass-fed beef, wild game, healthy oils, seeds, nuts, ancient grains, and fruits and vegetables. We cannot emphasize this enough. Chapter 14 will change your family's life.

Special diets. In addition to eating anti-inflammatory foods, two specific diet overhauls can be life-changing for the allergy sufferer. This certainly was the case for me, as these dietary changes were probably the most significant factor in resolving my asthma. Chapter 8 presents the details of a gluten-free, low-carb lifestyle, explaining how grain-based carbs increase inflammation and how gluten-sensitive people react to our nation's genetically modified wheat. Chapter 14 expands this advice to include all grains and milk products and describes how the "paleolithic" style of eating, along with fermented foods (with natural probiotics) can help heal inflammation and allergic disorders. We also suggest you eat organic, non–genetically modified (non-GMO) foods to maximize your family's return to health. Pages 202 through 206 offer details on how to clean up the diet.

Reducing environmental toxins. As you learned in the first chapter, chemicals and toxins increase allergies. We suggest you turn your home into a "green" house to avoid as many of those toxins as possible. From the household cleaning solutions and hygiene products you use to the furniture you buy and the food you eat, everything must be as organic and natural as possible. Achieving this change requires a lot of initial work, but it is fairly easy to maintain once you are on the right track. Numerous books and websites are available to guide you through this process, including several insightful guides put out by the Environmental Working Group (EWG.org).

Medications. Appropriate use of allergy and asthma medications can make life much happier for allergy sufferers. I find myself popping an oral antihistamine from time to time without chagrin. ICS inhalers and oral leukotriene inhibitors are also effective for reducing allergic response. Reliance upon chronic daily medication to control asthma doesn't really qualify as *resolution* of asthma, but it may be needed for a period to get the allergies under control.

Salt inhalation therapy. This treatment is gaining attention, and we believe it has merit. The theory stems from the ancient practice of spending prolonged periods in salt caves or taking in the salty air of the ocean shore to cure chronic respiratory ailments. One research study demonstrates the efficacy of salt inhalation therapy with regard to asthma. As previously mentioned, I found significant relief when I first started using a Himalayan crystal salt inhaler every day, and I still use this therapy on most days to maintain my lung health. These inhalers are available online and from some natural health care practitioners. You can also visit a facility that simulates a salt cave experience for more potent therapy (find one online).

Traditional Chinese medicine. Research has demonstrated that Chinese licorice root in combination with other herbal remedies may decrease inflammation and relax the muscles around the airways, thus providing asthma relief naturally. In addition, some research supports the efficacy of acupuncture and acupressure as legitimate treatments for asthma. Consider availing yourself of these approaches with a licensed practitioner who is knowledgeable in Chinese medicine.

Chiropractic and osteopathic care. We use chiropractic care for back pain and injuries in our families on a regular basis, but chiropractic and other manipulative medical approaches also claim to yield benefits in allergy prevention. As you read on page 11, part of the body's allergic response is mediated by the nervous system. Professional manipulation of the neck and spine can calm down these areas of the nervous system so that allergy sufferers don't react as strongly to allergens. This is worth pursuing for those who suffer from persistent symptoms.

Homeopathy. This practice uses tiny doses of remedies that match a person's body type and chemistry in an effort to reduce allergic responses. Under the care of an experienced practitioner, we have seen some patients respond well. But results are inconsistent, and some don't find relief from homeopathy. It is certainly safe to try, and some will find it worth the time and effort. See page 312 for more details.

Natural supplements. Various nutrient and antioxidant supplements reduce body inflammation and allergies, particularly high-dose fish oil supplementation, vitamin D, probiotics, and probiotic foods. Magnesium supplementation (about 250 milligrams two to four times daily under the care of a health care professional) may help relax constricted lung airways and help relieve an asthma attack. See page 298 for details.

NAET therapy. Described on page 26, this alternative medicine practice has some anecdotal support as an effective way to reduce allergy responses to specific allergens.

Allergy shots. If you have tried every possible allergy elimination measure and natural treatment but continue to have persistent asthma symptoms, it's time to consider allergy shots. These can reduce allergic sensitivity to a variety of asthma-inducing allergens, including dust mites, pollen, mold, pets, and others. Discuss this with your allergy specialist. See page 264 for more on allergy shots.

Sublingual immunotherapy. This newly approved treatment involves placing small allergen pills under the tongue every day to allow the immune system to become tolerant of the allergen. It is not approved for those with severe asthma because of a small risk of triggering a severe asthma attack. See page 264 for more information.

Don't give up on asthma. Keep working with your health care provider and complementary/alternative health care providers until you achieve the quality of life and active lifestyle you and your children deserve.

EVOLVING INHALER TECHNOLOGY

For decades many inhalers used a chemical called chlorofluoro-carbon (CFC) to propel the medication out of the inhaler as a mist. CFCs destroy the ozone layer, so these have been phased out and replaced by HFA inhalers, which use hydrofluoro-alkane instead. If your old inhaler is no longer available because of this reason, it may become available soon. Ask your doctor or pharmacist.

5

Eczema

Eczema, also known as atopic dermatitis, is a chronic allergic disorder that mainly involves the skin. Almost all cases begin in young children before the age of five. After the initial few years of problematic disease, a lot of children will show improvement later in childhood. Many will outgrow eczema completely, but some will have persistent disease throughout their adult years.

Of all the allergic disorders we see in our office, eczema is the most troublesome, for several reasons: First, eczema commonly begins at an age much younger than asthma and nasal allergies; it's always difficult to see three-month-olds suffering from persistently dry, irritated, itchy skin, with open sore patches from constant scratching. Second, infant eczema can be a harbinger of many years of allergic challenges to come; some with early eczema will go on to develop asthma and other allergies. Third, the mainstay of eczema therapy is topical steroid cream. Although steroid cream is effective and safe in appropriate courses, long-term steroid use isn't ideal. Fourth, eczema requires daily regimens and routines that take a lot of time and effort; these young patients, and their parents, must devote part of each day to eczema therapy, time that could be better spent laughing and playing together. And finally, some infants don't improve significantly despite aggressive testing and therapy, and those early years can be very tough for such babies.

That's the bad news. Now for some good news: Some cases of eczema resolve quite easily with some fairly simple steps. These are the cases in which the eczema is caused by one or two food allergies—and once the food is eliminated, the family can move on to better times. Those who don't find such an easy fix will face many challenges, and this chapter provides you with a detailed approach to doing everything you can to diagnose the cause and to eliminate the disorder.

IMMUNOLOGY AND GENETICS OF ECZEMA

Extensive research has been devoted to examining the skin, immune system, and genetics of those affected by eczema, and many details of the disorder have been carefully worked out. Here are some of the highlights:

Skin Inflammation

Virtually every type of immune blood cell is present in high numbers in the skin of affected individuals. These are a mix of acute and chronic inflammatory cells, indicating that eczema is an ongoing process that waxes and wanes. These cells secrete their cytokines (see page 8), which irritate the skin and draw more immune cells to the area. In addition, many with eczema have an overgrowth of staph bacteria on the skin that secrete more toxins and elevate the immune system's inflammatory reaction.

Allergic Flare-ups

Some cases of eczema are caused by food or environmental allergies. Exposure to these allergens causes the classic IgE allergic reaction described for other allergic disorders, which contributes to an already inflamed state within the skin.

Genetically Defective Skin

Eczema has a strong genetic component. About half of those who suffer from moderate to severe eczema have a mutation in what is called the FLG gene; this gene is responsible for producing filaggrin protein, which plays a crucial role in keeping moisture within the skin and maintaining proper pH. Those who have this mutation are also more likely to eventually develop asthma and other allergies. There are thought to be other genetic factors as well that have not yet been discovered.

The challenge with eczema is that it is not simply a matter of determining the offending allergen and eliminating it, as is the case with most other allergic disorders. Many with eczema have underlying genetically determined inflammatory tendencies that result in ongoing skin disease despite thorough elimination of the allergens. The hope for those with eczema is that the primary cause is a food allergy, the removal of which will resolve the disease and discomfort. If not, the focus should be put on proper skin care and using effective therapies to keep the eczema to a minimum.

SYMPTOMS OF ECZEMA

Virtually all infants and young children have a rash from time to time; this is a normal part of life. Eczema, however, has several distinct features that make it easily identifiable:

Dry, Irritated Patches

The basic eczema rash can be described as red, raised, itchy patches. Upon closer examination, the rash has some variation based on the stage of the disease:

Early stages. When eczema first occurs, or during sudden flares with chronic disease, the rash will appear as extremely itchy red bumps with scratched areas, some small blisters, and a small amount of moist secretions.

Middle stages. Once eczema has been present for a month or two, these severe areas will calm down from time to time into red, itchy patches that don't appear so angry and irritated.

Chronic eczema. Once the disease has been around for a while, the skin will thicken and the bumps will dry and harden. New flare-ups will occur from time to time, which start the process all over again.

Chronicity

Most harmless rashes come and go, but untreated eczema persists day after day, week after week, for months on end. Any rashes that come and go on their own are unlikely to be eczema.

Dry Skin

Those with eczema will have scattered patches of irritated skin, but underlying it all is a dryness over the entire body. Run your hand over the arms and legs of a child with eczema, and around the tummy and the back, and you will feel a prickly dryness throughout.

Itching

If there is one aspect of eczema that is certain, it is itching. Rashes that look like eczema but are not itchy are probably not eczema. This itchiness significantly interferes with sleep and quality of life for infants and children.

Location

Eczema has two distinct patterns that help confirm the diagnosis, and these depend on age:

Infants and toddlers. Eczema primarily affects the face, the scalp, and the outer surfaces of the arms and front surfaces of the legs (called the extensor surfaces of the extremities) in the younger years. However, this isn't always the case; some infants will develop the rash on the flexor surfaces of the arms and legs (the folds of the elbows and behind the knees). Wrists and ankles are also commonly affected.

Eczema almost never affects the diaper area, and the absence of rash (other than common diaper rash) in this location helps support the diagnosis.

Children two years of age and older and adults. In older age groups, eczema mainly appears on the flexor surfaces. All age groups may also suffer some rash on the chest, abdomen, and back as well, and a subgroup of people will develop rash around the eyes.

Doctors are well versed in diagnosing eczema; your primary care doctor should easily be able to identify the rash and help set you on the road to treatment and testing for allergies.

ALLERGY TESTING IN ECZEMA

Research has shown that about 35 percent of eczema cases in children are caused by food allergies. As you read above, a significant food allergy is the primary hope for resolution of the disorder. Therefore, this should be a key focus when eczema is first diagnosed; review the food allergy chapters to get yourself started. A small number of eczema cases are caused by environmental allergies like dust and pets, so these should be tested as well. The way we approach allergy diagnosis for eczema patients in our office depends on the age of onset and the infant's primary source of nutrition.

Breastfed Infants

Food allergy testing isn't very accurate in young infants. Instead, observational trials with food elimination are the most useful way to assess infant food allergies.

The most likely cause of young-infant eczema is from cow's milk protein passing through Mom's breast milk. Our first step with eczema babies, before any testing is done, is to have Mom eliminate all cow's milk products from her diet. See page 136 for a reminder on how to accomplish this, and Chapter 14 for how to eliminate the other top allergy foods. The eczema should improve within a few weeks if dairy is the culprit. Realize that an infant can develop these food allergies at any age; your baby may have previously seemed fine without any dietary restrictions, but don't let that prevent you from considering this factor now.

If dairy elimination doesn't do it, eggs should be next on your list, as an egg allergy has a particular connection to eczema in young children. After that come wheat and other gluten grains. If these restrictions don't fix the eczema, you should remove all of the top nine allergenic foods simultaneously: milk, wheat, eggs, soy, tree nuts, peanuts, fish, shellfish, and corn.

Formula-Fed Infants

Cow's milk–based infant formula is a likely cause in babies who are formula-fed. With your doctor's guidance, you should try a variety of infant formulas until you find one that the baby doesn't react to. It can take a few weeks for eczema to clear completely once the allergen is removed, but you should see some improvement within a week of changing a formula. Review page 136 in Chapter 7, "Milk Allergy and Sensitivity," for information on formula options.

Infants Six Months and Older

By six months of age, we consider allergy testing valuable enough to be worth the cost and trouble for infants in whom eczema has persisted despite elimination diets and formula changes. As you read in previous chapters, allergy testing is more accurate at two years of age. However, in cases of moderate to severe eczema, testing can reveal the allergic culprits during infancy. Your doctor can help you decide whether to do blood testing or see an allergist for skin testing.

Older Children and Adults

Any person with eczema who has not been tested for allergies deserves this evaluation. If you have had testing already but your eczema persists, repeat the testing every few years to rule out any new allergies. Food allergies are not the only possible culprit; rarely, pet, dust, or other inhalant allergies can trigger eczema, and eliminating contact with these factors can help significantly. See Chapter 13 for more information.

Other Tests to Rule Out Unusual Causes of Eczema

Most cases of eczema are really just eczema. Rarely, certain immune deficiency disorders can present with eczema-like rashes. Intestinal parasites, which are uncommon in the United States, can also trigger eczema. In consultation with your doctor, consider running the following tests to rule out these unusual causes of eczema-like rash:

CBC with differential. This complete blood count test examines all the present blood cell types and will reveal various types of immune disorders. It also tests for anemia (which is unrelated to eczema but is a valuable screening test in young kids). Perhaps the most useful part of the test, however, is that it measures the level of *eosinophils* (a type of white blood cell; see page 5). High eosinophils can be an indication of several problems, including intestinal parasites, eosinophilic disorders (see page 211), and hyper-IgE syndrome (see "Blood IgE level" below). Having high eosinophils is not specifically diagnostic of these disorders, but it is a useful test that should raise suspicion should a chronic rash be more than simple eczema.

Blood IgE level. Immunoglobulin E, as you learned on page 8, is the antibody that responds to allergens. A total IgE level is often included in blood allergy panels. Those with allergic disorders are expected to have an elevated level measuring in the hundreds. However, there is a rare type of immune disorder called *hyper-IgE syndrome,* which yields IgE levels of 2,000 or higher. High eosinophils are also usually present. Those with hyper-IgE usually have chronic skin infections and may have other recurrent infections like pneumonia and fungal infections. Proper diagnosis of this syndrome is complex and beyond the scope of this book. A full discussion can be found online on the Immune Deficiency Foundation's website, PrimaryImmune.org. Those with severe, persistent eczema should have an IgE blood level and CBC with differential test to rule out this disorder.

Stool test for parasites. Although it's uncommon, parasites can infect those living in developed countries. Even some harmless parasites, which don't cause any intestinal symptoms, can irritate the allergic branch of the immune system and trigger eczema rashes. A stool analysis is worth doing, particularly in those with high eosinophils and high IgE levels.

ONSET OF ECZEMA RIGHT AFTER INFANT VACCINATIONS

Some infants will experience their first flare of eczema right after one of the big rounds of vaccines at two, four, or six months of age. It isn't clear whether vaccines are the cause of such cases, as we have seen some unvaccinated infants develop eczema around this age as well. But vaccines do stimulate the immune system in an artificial manner. Furthermore, vaccines contain ingredients that can trigger allergic reactions, such as soy in the pneumococcal vaccine (given at two, four, six, and fifteen months of age) and egg in the flu vaccine (given at six and seven months and yearly thereafter) and the MMR vaccine (given at one and five years). There are also numerous chemical and germ components in vaccines, which a small percentage of infants will be sensitive to. It stands to reason that, although most infants handle vaccines without reactions, a small percentage will have a negative immune reaction that results in the stimulation of the allergic and inflammatory components of the immune system. For such babies, the disease protection afforded by vaccines may not be worth the ongoing negative immunological effects.

In our office, we postpone subsequent vaccines if an infant develops eczema during the weeks after a round of vaccines,

(continued)

especially if the reaction is severe. We do not resume vaccines until the eczema has subsided, and we avoid soy- and egg-containing vaccines until testing has ruled out those allergies. If the eczema remains moderate to severe for many months, you and your doctor will decide when the need to resume vaccines outweighs the risk of the eczema.

TREATING ECZEMA

Eczema therapy is complex and multifactorial. In addition to eliminating allergens, the skin must be properly cared for to minimize itching and inflammation. But eczema care is much more than skin deep; the whole body must be healthy to minimize eczema. Gut health is critical for a healthy immune and allergy system. Proper nutrition to reduce inflammation is key. The brain must be tended to as well, which means living a lifestyle that minimizes stress. In this section we focus on skin care, and be sure to read Chapter 14 as well, for tips on how proper nutrition and lifestyle can reduce allergies and inflammation.

Moisturize the Skin

The single most important factor in controlling eczema is to keep the skin moist. Numerous moisturizers are available, and each one claims to be the best; we have been happy with dozens of them over the years and do not have any favorite brands. You will likely try a variety of products until you find one that best suits you or your child. You may need to rotate the products you use throughout the year, as some may feel better during the hot and sweaty summer months and others may feel better during the cool, dry winter. Apply moisturizers liberally as many times each day as needed to keep the skin smooth and to prevent dryness. Here are some choices to help get you started:

Try basic moisturizing lotions and creams. You will find dozens of name-brand moisturizing products on the shelf of every drugstore. Your doctor will likely suggest some brands that he or she has found to work well, but you are welcome to try any on your own.

Try natural lotions and oils. We have found that natural moisturizers, available by searching online or at large health food stores, work just as well as those mentioned above, or for some people, even better—and they have the added advantage of being free of numerous chemical ingredients. Such products come as creams, lotions, oils, or thicker "butters." Effective ingredients include shea butter, cocoa butter, jojoba oil, and coconut oil. Because you will be applying such products on a daily basis, chemical-free is a safer choice.

Bathe long and daily. Doctors used to advise people with eczema to limit baths, as some soaps, shampoos, and hot water can irritate eczematous skin. It is now believed that soaking in a warm (not hot) bath without soap for fifteen minutes every day effectively hydrates the skin. Warm wet towel soaks can be applied to facial eczema, and hand or foot rashes can benefit from soaking in large containers of warm water if whole baths aren't needed. Drip dry when done, then gently pat away excess water; don't vigorously rub the skin dry, as this may irritate it. Apply moisturizer to damp skin to lock in the water.

Control humidity. For many with eczema, the dry winter months are the worst. But for some, hot, sweaty summers cause flare-ups. Keeping the humidity level in your home as steady as possible may minimize these swings. Buy a humidity gauge, and use humidifiers and dehumidifiers as needed to maintain humidity between 25 and 40 percent. Air conditioning will also help during the summer, and be careful not to overheat your home during the winter, as this dries out the air.

Drink more water. It sounds so simple, but increasing water intake provides more moisture for the skin. Some kids are hesitant if you push them, but try to model copious drinking from water bottles throughout the day so the habit will catch on with your kids.

OIL THE SKIN AND BODY

When we say oil, we are actually referring to the healthy omega-3 oils in fish. Research has shown that these healthy fats help reduce eczema and other allergic disorders. Breastfeeding moms should enjoy plenty of fish in their diet, especially wild salmon, and take a fish-oil supplement, so that their baby's dry, irritated skin can benefit from the soothing effects of healthy fish fats through Mom's breast milk. Infants with eczema can also be given fish oil supplements directly under the supervision of your doctor. Make wild salmon one of baby's first protein foods by eight months of age. See page 291 for more research on the benefits of salmon and omega-3 supplements.

Avoid Skin Irritants

Many things in life irritate the skin; for those with eczema this is doubly true. Here are some key items to pay close attention to:

Take care with your laundry. Say good-bye to that yummy baby smell of fabric softeners and the fresh spring scent of your laundry detergent; these chemicals are not friendly to those with eczema. Dryer sheets are also out. Use unscented detergents designed for sensitive skin, and double-rinse the wash to remove as much soap as possible.

Dress right. Some people are sensitive to synthetic clothing or wool and find that organic cotton is best. Dress infants and young children in lightweight, loose-fitting long sleeves and pants to reduce scratching of irritated extremities.

Bathe right. In addition to long soaks in a warm bath, be sure to use the right bath products. Plain soap can dry the skin; unscented moisturizing soap may be best for most people. Use chemical-free, organic shampoos. For those with scalp eczema, tea tree oil shampoo or a tar-based shampoo may reduce scalp irritation.

Another factor that contributes to eczema is the calcium, chlorine, and other chemicals in bathwater. New research shows that hard water raises the risk of infant eczema five-fold! Buy a water filter for your shower head (available online and in hardware stores) that removes these irritants and softens the water, and use the shower head to fill the bath for your long soaks. Whole-house water filters are also available, but at quite a price.

Reduce scratching. Keep fingernails cut short. Mittens and socks may need to be worn at night to limit a child's ability to scratch with her finger- and toenails.

Choose the right suntan lotion. Use natural, chemical-free lotions; PABA is one ingredient that can irritate eczema.

Take care with swimming pools. Chlorine is not your friend. If you, or a family member, are a frequent swimmer, try to find a salt-water pool for your routine recreation. When you do swim in a chlorinated pool, rinse afterward in fresh water as soon as possible.

Medicated Therapy

Virtually everyone with eczema will need medical therapy from time to time. The mainstay of prescription therapy is topical steroids. Antihistamines are also useful, and some nonsteroidal anti-inflammatory therapies can bring relief. Here are the options on which your doctor will advise you:

Topical steroids. Although the word *steroid* is scary to most parents, these creams, lotions, and ointments bring much-needed relief and are very safe when used appropriately. Mild, over-the-counter hydrocortisone can be safely used for long periods. Stronger prescriptions, which are graded on a scale of one through seven (group 1 being the most potent), should be used with care and supervised by a doctor. The higher the potency, the better it will work, but the stronger groups are more likely to cause side effects (see below). We strongly advise against obtaining repeat refills of potent prescriptions without seeing your doctor.

Steroid groups 6 and 7 can be safely used for months at a time. The midrange groups, 3 to 5, can be used for several weeks if needed. The highest-potency groups, 1 and 2, should be reserved for short-term use (a few weeks at most) to bring severe flare-ups under control. A common practice is for a doctor to prescribe a strong cream to be used for a set period, followed by a milder cream to keep the eczema at bay. Be sure you understand which group your prescription steroids fall into and how long your doctor advises you to use them.

Side effects are extremely rare with the mild groups and are uncommon with the moderate ones. When negative effects do occur, the most likely is a thinning of the skin or a loss of pigmentation; less common effects include stretch marks, blood vessel blemishes (called telangiectasia or purpura), acne, and skin infections. Chronic use on the face can lead to worsened inflammation around the mouth. The face, armpits, and groin are particularly sensitive to side effects, and strong formulations should be avoided in these areas.

Nonsteroidal prescription creams. Several brand-name products have recently been formulated to treat eczema without the use of steroids. They tend to be less effective, but they are a welcome alternative to chronic steroids for those in whom they work well. Brand names include Atopiclair, Eletone, EpiCeram, and MimyX. These are made from a variety of oils, fats, and other compounds that reduce inflammation and promote skin healing. Your doctor will advise you on these options.

Immune-suppressing creams. Tacrolimus and pimecrolimus are two relatively new prescription therapies that are somewhat controversial. They work by suppressing the immune system (through a mechanism different from that of steroids), thus decreasing the allergic inflammation in the skin. However, early studies showed that these creams create a very slight risk of lymphoma. Follow-up research has demonstrated that this is not true, but this worry has limited the use of these creams by many doctors. We have seen these creams work well in our few patients who have tried it, and we encourage you to consider it if other therapies are not working well.

Antihistamines. These useful allergy medications, discussed on page 41, are essential for those with uncontrolled eczema who need relief from the daily itch. Sedating ones, like diphenhydramine (brand name Benadryl), are ideal for overnight use, and nondrowsy options can be used during the day. Those with severe disease may benefit from chronic antihistamine therapy, under the guidance of their doctor.

Moist wraps. Under the guidance of an allergy specialist or dermatologist, you can wrap severely affected areas in wet dressings or clothing. This helps lock in moisture. These dressings can also be placed over medicated creams to improve absorption. Overuse, however, can damage the skin, so this should only be done according to a doctor's instructions.

Natural anti-inflammatory creams. Several herbal treatments are known to reduce inflammation and itching, including primrose oil, chamomile, calendula, and aloe vera. Try these as a way to minimize medicated therapy; they work well for some.

Keep Bacteria at Bay

A particular challenge for those with eczema is colonization with staph bacteria. Studies show that almost everyone with eczema has these bacteria growing within their eczema lesions, whereas very few people with healthy skin are infected. Staph bacteria secrete toxins that exacerbate inflammation in the skin, causing the eczema lesions to worsen. However, continuous use of antibiotics can lead to resistance and worsen the infection as well. Periodic courses of oral or topical antibiotics, under the careful guidance of your doctor, are appropriate for skin infections (angry red flare-ups with moist or crusty drainage) and should help reduce severe flare-ups of the eczema too. Your doctor may also suggest periodic skin cleansing with an antiseptic cleanser (chlorhexidine) or diluted bleach baths. Prescription nasal antibiotic ointment can be used to eliminate staph from the nose, which is a common source of this infection. Manuka honey from New Zealand, available in most health food stores, is an effective natural topical antibiotic for skin infections; we have seen it work well in our office in place of antibiotics. Fungal skin infections can also periodically flare; these can be identified by your doctor and treated with antifungal cream.

Anti-inflammatory Diet

Diet changes directed by positive allergy test results should improve eczema. In addition, following our general dietary approaches to reducing allergy and inflammation detailed in Chapter 14 can improve eczema, even if all food allergy testing is normal. Furthermore, some infants, children, and adults will respond well to low-carbohydrate dietary changes (eliminating grains and dairy) as described on page 303. In our practice, those who successfully incorporate our nutritional advice do best.

Allergy Shots

Some research has shown that immunotherapy for dust mite allergy in those with eczema can help reduce the condition. Discuss this option with your allergist, particularly if your child tests allergic to dust mites. See page 264 for more information.

6

Food Allergies and Sensitivities: Overview of Symptoms and Testing

Food allergies have become an increasingly common challenge for parents and children today. Some studies reveal that the incidence of food allergies has tripled in the past twenty years, and that they now affect over 10 percent of the American population. Researchers aren't certain why such a rise has occurred. We suspect various factors are involved, as discussed on page 13. A primary contributor to food allergies may be the food itself, or what our modern society has done to it. Genetically modified organisms (GMOs) in our food supply may change how the immune system reacts to common foods. Hormones and antibiotics in our meats and dairy products likely play a role as well, as do pesticides and other chemicals. These environmental factors literally alter how our genetic makeup responds to food, and for some of us, that response is an allergic one.

A CLOSER LOOK AT THE IMMUNE SYSTEM'S ALLERGIC (AND NONALLERGIC) RESPONSES TO FOOD

In Chapters 3 and 4 we've described how allergens trigger nasal allergies and asthma specifically in the nose and lungs. Allergic reactions to foods, however, can affect every body organ, and can follow several different immune and nonimmune pathways:

IgE-Mediated Food Allergy

In this straightforward allergic reaction, a person's immune system develops IgE antibodies against a food protein upon first exposure (and there's usually no noticeable reaction). These antibodies are attached to mast cells and basophils in the mucous lining of the nose, mouth, lungs, GI tract, and eyes, as well as in the bloodstream and various body organs. When these IgE antibodies come into contact with the allergic food again, the IgE causes each immune cell to release its histamines, leukotrienes, prostaglandins, and tryptase enzymes (see page 8), which trigger swelling, increased mucus secretion, and inflammation, and draw more allergic immune cells to the area. This response can also travel through the bloodstream and reach other body systems that have no contact with the food. For example, a person who is severely allergic to peanuts will experience some itching and tingling in the mouth and throat as the peanuts are chewed up and swallowed. The stomach and intestines will also react with discomfort and possible diarrhea. The allergic response travels quickly through the bloodstream to cause other organs to join in the reaction: the skin reacts with hives and itching, the lungs react with wheezing, the nose and throat may congest and swell, and even the major blood vessels can dilate and cause a fall in blood pressure and the resulting shock. Less severe allergic reactions may be restricted to only one body system, such as chronic nasal congestion from milk allergy, for example. The degree and symptoms of allergic reaction are unique to each individual and are fairly unpredictable. Such variations in allergic response with IgE-mediated food allergies are probably genetically determined, but we don't fully understand why and how this varies so widely from one allergy sufferer to the next.

Non IgE-Mediated Food Allergy

Some food allergies trigger an allergic type of immune reaction, but not via the IgE antibody pathway. These include celiac disease (severe gluten allergy generated via IgA antibodies), food protein–induced enterocolitis syndrome (or FPIES, in which T lymphocytes react directly to certain food proteins), and eosinophilic gastrointestinal disorders (like eosinophilic esophagitis, an allergic reaction via eosinophils instead of IgE). These will be explained in further detail in their respective sections or chapters.

IgG-mediated food allergy is a new field of study that many integrative medical practitioners have begun to explore. Blood tests are available to measure the level of IgG antibodies for almost every food. Patients can have hundreds of foods tested in just one blood draw. As you read on page 23, the theory holds that IgG reactions to food reflect a delayed and chronic immune reaction to that food, which can have a negative effect on a person's health. Eliminating such foods for an extended period may result in improved health. We believe that this type of testing may have merit, and it is a viable option for those with chronic immune, allergic, or developmental disorders. We do acknowledge, however, that research to verify the accuracy of this testing is lacking.

Food Intolerance or Sensitivity

These interchangeable terms refer to food reactions that don't involve the allergic pathway of the immune system. Examples include IgG-mediated food allergy (described above), which some refer to as food sensitivity, lactose intolerance (inability to digest milk sugar, or lactose, which results in intestinal symptoms), non-celiac gluten sensitivity (a milder form of gluten sensitivity that yields normal celiac disease test results), hyperactivity from sugar overload, behavioral challenges caused by chemicals like food coloring and preservatives, wheezing caused by sensitivity to sulfites in wine, and brain excitability caused by MSG. Some foods affect the body in a negative way due to their chemical nature, and this can present itself via nonallergic behavioral or neurological symptoms. Intolerance or sensitivity reactions are not considered true allergies, but they warrant just as much attention. More details on how these chemicals affect us will follow in Chapter 9.

Regardless of the mechanism, food reactions have a profound effect on health, development, and quality of life. In this chapter we explore the symptoms of food allergy and sensitivity, and how to begin the process of tracking down which unknown food is causing chronic and bothersome symptoms. In subsequent chapters, we will present more specific details on common and uncommon food allergy and sensitivity syndromes.

SYMPTOMS OF FOOD ALLERGY OR SENSITIVITY

Sometimes food reactions are obvious and immediate, and other times they are subtle and develop gradually. Food allergy reactions (IgE and non-IgE mediated) will cause classic allergic signs on the skin and in the respiratory tract and the gut. Food sensitivities, on the other hand, tend to trigger intestinal, behavioral, and neurological reactions, as well as some subtle skin rashes. Here are signs that suggest your child may have a food allergy or sensitivity:

Rash

The skin is one organ that loves to declare allergic reactions. Here are some of the symptoms you may see:

Hives. These itchy, raised welts are typically white in the center with a surrounding light red color. They come in all shapes and sizes, and several may coalesce into large patches of raised skin. They fade quickly (within an hour or two), only to pop up elsewhere on the body. Hives occur because the histamine released under the skin during an allergic reaction draws fluid and other immune cells into the area. Treatment with an antihistamine (see page 41) usually reduces or resolves the hives within fifteen to thirty minutes.

Eczema rash. While hives are the primary rash seen with immediate food allergy reactions, eczema-type rashes are a common sign of chronic food allergies. Chapter 5 explores eczema in detail, but it is mentioned here as a significant sign that food allergies need to be explored.

Other rashes. Some kids will show redness on the face and cheeks or around the anus. Others will develop chronic fine pimply bumps on the face, upper arms, and legs (called keratosis pilaris). Red ears may also be a sign of sensitivity.

Gastrointestinal Symptoms

The gut is a window into our health. If stools aren't soft, normal-shaped logs (outside of infancy), something is likely wrong. Food allergies will often trigger chronic irritation in the gut that results in abnormal stools. Here are some key manifestations to watch for:

Infants with runny, mucusy stools. Healthy stools of breastfed infants should look like yellow cottage cheese or gourmet seedy mustard. Those who are formula-fed may have darker yellow or brown mushy stools. There should be no mucus or drippy liquid. Sorry to get graphic, but this is important information.

Infants with severe spitting up or vomiting. Most infants spit up their breast milk or formula on a daily basis. Those who are happy and thriving probably don't have any underlying medical condition. But for those with severe symptoms, a food allergy or sensitivity should be ruled out. In addition, problematic spitting up can be a sign of gastroesophageal reflux disease (GERD), which may or may not be related to a food or formula sensitivity. Even more serious, eosinophilic esophagitis (EoE or EE) is a variation of GERD that is directly related to severe food allergy. Finally, food protein–induced enterocolitis syndrome (FPIES) is a newly recognized disorder that causes severe vomiting when certain baby foods are introduced. More on these conditions in Chapter 10.

"Toddler diarrhea." We put this term in quotes to make a point. Toddlers shouldn't have diarrhea. Yet the pediatric medical community has coined this term as a "normal" phase that many toddlers go through. Most pediatricians will try to reassure parents not to worry about runny or mucusy stools because such stools are common during these years. If it's common, it must be normal, right? Wrong. What *is* common is food allergy, and when do toddlers start eating some of the most allergic foods? After age one. In our practice, we consider toddler diarrhea a medical condition that deserves investigation until it is solved. The most common cause of toddler diarrhea is cow's milk allergy or lactose intolerance, followed by gluten sensitivity. More on this in Chapters 7 and 8.

Constipation. The opposite of diarrhea, this uncomfortable condition is also often caused by cow's milk sensitivity. For some kids, cow's milk (and, less commonly, gluten foods) can have a chemical effect on the gut that slows down colon contractions and causes chronic constipation. See page 158 for more information.

Recurrent abdominal pain, gas, or bloating. Sometimes a child's stools seem healthy, but he complains of chronic pain, passes excessive gas, and has a belly that looks like he's got something growing inside it. Investigating food allergy or sensitivity is important in such children.

Respiratory and Nasal Symptoms

You were introduced to nasal allergies and asthma in the first chapters. Although environmental inhalant allergens are more likely to be the primary triggers, food allergy should also be considered, especially in the early years of life.

Chronic runny nose or congestion. Milk allergy is the most common food trigger for these symptoms. Consider cow's milk proteins passing through breast milk or in infant formula if your infant has these chronic symptoms. Watch for these signs when introducing cow's milk after age one. Soy protein allergy is a less common possibility.

Chronic chest congestion or cough. Milk allergy, again, is the most likely food culprit for chronic chest symptoms, followed by soy.

Recurrent Infections

Food allergies may increase nasal and lung congestion, leading to sinus, ear, or chest infections. If your child is repeatedly ill, consider food allergy as a possible cause. The classic scenario we see in our office is a two-year-old who has had five ear infections in the past year, and no one has thought about eliminating cow's milk from the diet. Food sensitivity, especially to gluten, can lower the immune system and contribute to these infections as well.

Behavioral Challenges

Excessive temper tantrums, hyperactivity, and defiant behavior can be caused by food sensitivity. Food chemicals are the primary culprits: food coloring, artificial sweeteners, and preservatives. Refined sugar should also be suspect in these scenarios. And again, cow's milk and gluten sensitivity can cause such behaviors. We see many children heading toward the label of a behavioral disorder who become new kids when their diet is cleaned up. The chapters that follow discuss how to eliminate these foods, and pages 202 through 210 describe how to eat chemical-free.

Infant Colic

Classic pediatric teaching holds that colic doesn't have a dietary cause; it is simply digestive and neurological immaturity that will resolve over time. Most modern pediatricians, including those in our practice, would beg to differ. We have seen countless cases of colic resolve when food allergies or sensitivities are identified. More on this in Chapter 10.

Language and Other Developmental Delays

As developmental delays continue to rise among American children, finding treatable causes has become a primary goal in our pediatric practice. One such cause that we continually find as we work with these families is gluten and cow's milk sensitivity. In some susceptible children, these foods are improperly digested into proteins that mimic morphine-like compounds, which depress brain and gut function. See page 158 for more on this theory.

TESTING FOR FOOD ALLERGY AND SENSITIVITY

As you read in Chapter 2, several tests are available to evaluate food allergy and sensitivity: skin tests, IgE food allergy panels, IgG food sensitivity panels, and some alternative methods. Your doctor will guide you in deciding when testing is necessary and which form the testing should take. Numerous factors should be considered when choosing if, when, and how to test:

Age

Infants less than 1 year. Allergy testing is not very accurate at this young age. An infant may be allergic to cow's milk, for example, but tests may not reveal any reaction. On the other hand, positive results on a test are very reliable. Testing should be reserved for infants with allergies that don't improve when the more common allergens are eliminated for a time.

Young children. Blood testing is more easily tolerated for most young kids, compared to the multiple small pricks of skin testing. A wide array of allergens can be tested with just one blood draw.

Older children and adults. Skin testing with an allergist may have a slight advantage in accuracy, so as soon as a child is old enough to tolerate a skin testing procedure (see page 18), this may be the best route to take. If you prefer to have your primary care doctor order blood allergy testing, that is also a useful place to start.

Type of Symptoms

Your choice of testing may depend upon the type of symptoms you are evaluating.

Common allergic symptoms. If you are trying to find foods that are causing primary symptoms of allergy, such as hives, eczema, or nasal or respiratory symptoms, a blood IgE panel or a skin test are useful choices.

Behavioral symptoms. Blood tests for food sensitivity (IgG food panel and testing for gluten intolerance) may be the best place to begin to determine which foods may be causing behavioral reactions. However, reliability of IgG testing isn't certain. Observation during food elimination and reintroduction trials is a more reliable method of tracking down the culprits. More on this later.

Recurrent infections. To examine which foods may be responsible for triggering recurrent infections, several modes of testing may be useful. IgE food blood tests or skin tests can help determine which foods are causing increased nasal and respiratory congestion (which can lead to infection), and IgG food sensitivity tests and gluten intolerance tests (see page 22) can assess which foods may be suppressing the immune system.

Gastrointestinal symptoms. These can be caused by both food allergy and sensitivity; blood testing for IgE and IgG food reactions, along with gluten intolerance, is the appropriate approach.

Severity of Symptoms

Before you embark on expensive and invasive testing, assess whether or not the allergy symptoms warrant testing. Mild symptoms that are only intermittent may not. Those with mild symptoms might not register any positive results on testing anyway. Save the testing procedures for later, if allergies persist or worsen.

Duration of Symptoms

If symptoms have just recently begun, you may be more likely to deduce the cause without tests. For example, perhaps you just introduced a new food group, such as milk for your toddler.

Those who have had symptoms for many years, on the other hand, are less likely to realize the cause, and probably require testing.

Seasonal Timing of Symptoms

If your symptoms keep recurring year after year at the same time, and you enjoy much of the year without symptoms, you likely have pollen or mold allergies; you don't necessarily need food allergy testing. If symptoms don't follow a predictable seasonal pattern, and persist much of the year, tests will be more helpful.

Observation Without Testing

Sometimes you can deduce the cause of allergy or sensitivity symptoms without testing. Food testing isn't very accurate in young children, so it may not be the most appropriate first step. Here are some common scenarios we see in the office that deserve a trial of elimination for the most likely food culprits before resorting to tests:

Infant colic or GERD. Colic and reflux should be approached as a food allergy or sensitivity through Mom's breast milk, or a formula allergy/sensitivity, until proven otherwise. Yet we rarely resort to testing these young babies. The best "tests" are eliminating the most likely foods from Mom's diet (cow's milk and gluten top the list) or making formula changes. IgE skin or blood testing is saved for those whose symptoms persist for several months. See Chapter 10 for more information on how to solve colic and GERD.

Infant and child eczema. The same goes for eczema. Eliminate suspected food allergens first, then rely on skin or blood IgE testing and gluten testing for persistent cases.

Infant and child nasal and lung allergies. These are uncommon, but when they do occur they are quite troublesome. Cow's milk products are again the most likely allergic culprit. Household inhalant allergies (dust, mold, pets) should also be considered. Eventual IgE allergy testing may be helpful if elimination steps don't solve the problem.

Infant and child intestinal symptoms. Cow's milk products should be the first to go. If there's no change, then go gluten-free. If symptoms persist, consider nonallergic causes (see Chapter 10). Food IgE allergy and IgG sensitivity testing and gluten intolerance testing can eventually be done.

Toddler and child behavioral problems. Go off cow's milk first. If that doesn't help, go gluten-free. You can see this is a common theme, as these are the two most likely foods to cause problems in children (review page 113 to remind yourself why this is). If challenges persist, IgG food sensitivity and gluten testing should be done.

Recurrent ear and/or sinus infections. We find that cow's milk allergy is a common contributor to ear infections, frequent colds, and sinus infections. Don't bother testing just yet. Eliminate dairy and see how your child does. Food IgE allergy testing can be done if problems persist.

Asthma. Once a child is diagnosed with asthma (lung allergy symptoms persist or recur enough for a diagnosis), thorough IgE allergy testing should be done (either blood or skin tests). Don't just keep guessing at the allergies.

NORMAL TEST RESULTS MEANS NO ALLERGY OR SENSITIVITY, RIGHT?

Wrong. Allergy tests *may* show a positive reaction to an allergen if the person is allergic, but they may not. If someone has an obvious allergic reaction to a food or other allergen, and that reaction is seen again with repeated exposure, that person is considered allergic. Testing does not confirm (or negate) that fact. The same is true with food sensitivities; if a negative reaction to food occurs on a consistent basis, and the reaction subsides when the food is avoided, that person *is* sensitive to that food, regardless of test results.

We see a common scenario in which patients are misled. It happens when a child or adult with obvious allergies gets tested by a doctor, the tests all come back normal, and the doctor tells them they don't have allergies. This also occurs with food sensitivities; someone suspected of gluten sensitivity gets tested and has normal results, and the doctor declares that the person is not gluten-sensitive.

A more correct way to interpret negative (or normal) allergy and sensitivity test results is to simply say that the test did not reveal for us what you are sensitive or allergic to, but based on your symptoms you *are* sensitive or allergic to something. Let's keep exploring possible causes and consider eliminating the most likely food culprits to observe what happens.

Component Food Allergy Blood Testing

This is a new technology that may help predict the likelihood of future reactions. ImmunoCAP is the first lab to develop this technology for peanuts, eggs, and milk; in the future, testing for other foods may become available, and other labs will likely offer such tests. Component testing measures the immune reaction to specific proteins within the foods instead of the whole food. Results can predict whether a person will react only to raw forms of the food (but will tolerate cooked forms), how severe the reaction is likely to be, and whether or not the person is likely to outgrow the allergy. This information will help you understand how careful you have to be with these three foods. Ask your doctor about component testing, and see the specific sections of Chapters 7 and 9 on milk, peanut, and egg allergies for more details on each test.

Oral Food Challenge Test

To make a diagnosis in years past, doctors relied on parent reports of reactions to food, along with allergy testing. New guidelines are calling for doctors to make more accurate diagnoses, as a food allergy diagnosis has a significant impact on a patient's life for years or decades to come. Positive allergy tests alone may not be enough to confirm a diagnosis because some people show an IgE antibody response to a food when tested, yet may not mount any observable allergic reaction in real life when eating the food. This phenomenon is called sensitization; a person may have IgE against a particular food, but that IgE won't trigger the immune cascade that results in symptoms. Those who are sensitized but don't exhibit symptoms of allergy are considered *not* allergic to that food.

To clarify the diagnosis, allergists will often perform an oral food challenge (OFC) test in the office. The patient will refrain from eating the suspected food for a prescribed number of weeks, during which they should be off antihistamine medications and should be relatively symptom-free. The food is consumed in gradually increasing amounts over an hour in the office, and the patient is observed for reaction. An allergic response confirms the diagnosis, and no reaction means the patient is sensitized but not necessarily allergic.

Oral food challenge testing is primarily useful in confirming immediate allergic reactions to food, but it certainly isn't practical in assessing chronic behavioral or intestinal reactions. Some allergy specialists may be too quick to dismiss a possible allergy when a patient doesn't demonstrate a reaction in their office. In addition, if a person has had an obvious and clear anaphylactic reaction after exposure to a likely allergic food, replaying this scenario and risking another anaphylactic reaction may not be necessary. Such tests should only be performed if truly needed.

PREVENTING FOOD ALLERGIES

Every new parent wants to prevent food allergies in their children, particularly if such allergies are already present in the family. You can take steps that will make a significant difference:

Extended Breastfeeding

We know for certain that breastfeeding helps prevent all allergic disorders, and the longer a child is breastfed, the better. American health policy makers recommend breastfeeding for at least a year, and world health leaders advise two years or more. We agree with the latter. Also, research shows that if gluten is introduced while an infant is still breastfeeding, the risk of that infant's eventually developing celiac disease (severe gluten allergy) is reduced. Furthermore, new research shows that continuing to breast feed for three or more months after cow's milk is introduced to a child (usually recommended after age one) reduces the risk of milk allergy and other food allergies. Immune components in breast milk help a child's gut learn to tolerate allergenic foods.

Mothers with Food Allergies

Women who have a particular food allergy are naturally going to avoid that food. This includes avoidance during pregnancy and breastfeeding. If the allergy is moderate to severe, we agree.

However, there is a drawback to this practice overall: it means that the developing infant won't be exposed to this particular food either in the womb or through Mom's breast milk. Food protein exposures in the early years actually help an infant's immune system become tolerant of such foods. Understandably, a mom with a moderate to severe allergy must avoid that food, and by default, the infant won't be exposed until he or she begins to eat the food directly. However, if a mom's food allergy or sensitivity is *mild,* it may be in the baby's best interest for Mom to eat the food periodically during pregnancy and breastfeeding, so that the baby's immune system gets some exposure. Some research shows that women who periodically eat the top allergic foods, such as peanuts, wheat, and dairy, during pregnancy actually reduce their child's chance of developing food allergies. Maternal cow's milk avoidance during breast feeding has been shown to increase the risk of later milk allergy in the child.

If Mom's allergy is moderate to severe, she may be inclined to avoid giving that food to her children as well. It may be better, however, to allow some careful exposure at the appropriate age (see "Introducing Foods at the Right Age," below). If the allergy is genetically programmed into the child, the age of first exposure may not matter; the allergy may happen regardless of what you do. But if the genetic component is not there, or the genetic risk is borderline, early exposure may prevent the allergy. Most research shows that delayed introduction of allergenic foods into the diet raises the risk of later allergy. The research isn't completely clear on this yet—but the old advice to completely avoid giving any family-allergic foods to children is no longer considered appropriate in all cases.

Fathers or Siblings with Food Allergies

If Dad or another child in the family has the allergy, the natural inclination may be to avoid that food in every subsequent child.

Instead, Mom should consume these foods during pregnancy and while breastfeeding, and she should carefully introduce the foods at the age-appropriate times (see below) to create tolerance in the child. However, stop the foods if and when any reactions occur.

Introducing Foods at the Right Age

We are going to let you in on a little secret: doctors don't know everything about everything. And if there's one area about which we *really* aren't certain, it's food introduction. There are many different ideas about what to introduce to a baby, how, and when, but no one really knows for sure because very little comparative research has been done to examine various feeding theories. We aren't completely ignorant, however. Here is the information that we *do* know (and what we think we know), which you can rely on as you choose the best way to introduce your baby to food:

When to start. Interestingly, some research shows that starting foods at four months helps prevent allergies, and other research shows that waiting until six months or later is better. So who's right? Most experts go with the six-month mark, and we agree. Some families with multiple food allergies are inclined to delay foods even longer, up to a year. Because breast milk provides all of a baby's necessary nutrition for the first year, foods aren't technically needed; delaying solids is, therefore, safe. But research hasn't proven that such a delay provides any protective benefits either, and some gluten research shows that delaying past seven months may actually increase later risk of gluten allergy.

What to start. The classic advice is to start with rice cereal and a few other bland foods like bananas, sweet potatoes, and applesauce. This idea, however, has no scientific basis. The reality is that a baby can start on pretty much *any* fruit and vegetable (avocados are our favorite). Some think veggies should go before fruits, but that hasn't been proven. Rice cereal has little nutritional value and might not be the healthiest first food because it is high in carbohydrates; as such, we have moved away from recommending it.

Spacing out first foods. When introducing foods, start with one food at a time, every few days, for the first few weeks to watch for allergic reactions. If you don't see any allergic signs in the first month, you don't have to be so careful in the months that follow; your baby can enjoy any new food at any time without worrying about spacing.

Moving forward. Between six and nine months, a baby can enjoy any fruit and vegetable. And it doesn't all have to be pureed. Let your baby hold and gnaw on whole fruits and veggies; this sends the message that food is natural and comes in many shapes, sizes, textures, and flavors. A baby's food should not come out of a pouch or jar; whole foods that come wrapped fresh in Mother Nature's natural peeling are probably best. Cereals are okay but aren't nutritionally necessary. When you do choose a cereal, use healthier grains like quinoa, amaranth, hemp, and other whole, natural grains. Since the food isn't required for nutrition yet (breast milk is complete nutrition for at least the first year), it doesn't matter how much baby swallows. Food should simply be fun.

At nine months a baby's diet can expand to include all meats, fish, eggs, legumes, nut butters, berries, and pretty much anything. In fact, the only food that we know babies shouldn't eat until after one year is honey, which can cause infant botulism. Some argue that we should not feed peanut and shellfish until one year as well, but research isn't certain on this. But virtually all experts agree that when a baby turns one year old, everything is fair game; there are no absolute food restrictions once that first birthday is past.

Allergenic foods. Here are some general guidelines on when you can safely start the top eight allergenic foods. Some research, as you will read below, supports introducing these at earlier ages. If any of these specific food allergies run in the family, ask your doctor before introducing them:

- Dairy: Cheese and yogurt are okay at nine months; cow's milk can be given at twelve months.
- Wheat: This can be started at nine months, but don't overdo it. Give a wide variety of grains (quinoa, amaranth, hemp, oat, wheat, rice, corn) so that baby isn't overloaded with only one type. Don't give baby too much bread, cereal, pasta, or other grain foods; a small serving every other day or so is appropriate. For families with celiac disease (severe wheat/gluten allergy), some research suggests that introduction around six months is better to induce immune tolerance (see page 163).
- Peanuts: Typical advice is to wait on peanuts until close to one year of age. However, as you will read in the peanut allergy section on page 189, countries that introduce peanut butter early (around six months) have much lower rates of peanut allergy. Nine months may be okay.
- Tree nuts: You can safely introduce these in the form of nut butters around nine months of age.
- Fish: This healthy food should be started around nine months.
- Shellfish: Delay these until one year as a precaution, since they aren't really a necessary food for infants.
- Eggs: These can be given at nine months of age.
- Soy: Soy foods, in moderation, can be started at nine months of age.

These are just general guidelines; adjustments can be made, with your doctor's advice, to suit your family's needs. Further research will provide better guidelines in years to come. Already, some studies published last year revealed some interesting findings:

- Breastfeeding for less than nine and a half months increased the risk of asthma.
- Early introduction of cow's milk (at an average of two months of age) increased the risk of eczema.
- Starting cereals made from corn, rice, millet, and buckwheat (which are, interestingly, gluten-free) by four months increased eczema, whereas starting a gluten cereal (wheat, oat, rye, or barley) by five and a half months actually lowered the risk of nasal allergies, eczema, and asthma.
- Giving eggs before eleven months lowered asthma, nasal allergy, and eczema.
- Starting fish between six and twelve months helped prevent allergies and asthma, whereas giving fish before six months, and delaying it until after twelve months, increased asthma risk.

Diversify. Research shows that a more diverse diet in the first year of life reduces the risk of asthma and food allergies. Offer a wide variety instead of sticking to only baby's favorite few foods.

Stay clear of "kids' menu" foods. Kids love chicken nuggets, mac and cheese, pizza, grilled cheese sandwiches, and French fries. We recommend you steer clear of these foods at home during the toddler years because kids tend to get so hooked on them that they shun many other foods. The overload of wheat and dairy in these foods, not to mention the carbs, isn't good for anybody. Shape your child's taste buds with healthy foods to create proper eating habits from an early age.

Stay clear of gimmick toddler snacks. You will notice a variety of toddler snacks on the shelf of every grocery store, even health food stores. Veggie puffs, fruit chews, melt-in-your-mouth yogurt bites, and pouches filled with every possible fruit or veggie imaginable. While there is nothing inherently unhealthy about such foods, we worry they may interfere with shaping children's tastes for natural foods. Sure, children love them, but children love candy too; that doesn't mean we let them have it every day. Staying committed to feeding only fresh, natural, unprocessed foods to infants and toddlers may better shape their taste buds for the natural antiallergy and anti-inflammatory foods we promote in Chapter 14.

Allergy research is constantly evolving, so if your family has a history of food allergies, it's always good to ask your doctor for the latest information.

ELIMINATING SENSITIVE AND ALLERGIC FOODS

You have observed your child's (and perhaps your own) symptoms of food allergy or sensitivity, you have eliminated some common food allergens as an initial trial, and perhaps you have had allergy testing to pinpoint the specific food allergens. Now you are ready to move forward, full steam ahead, with changing your child's and family's diet to accommodate the allergies and sensitivities. This is a big step, and it can be a daunting one at first. But it will change the course of your family's health for the better. This chapter is just an introduction to get you started down the right path. In the chapters that follow, we walk you through scenarios for each food allergy or sensitivity in more detail. Use our information to complement the advice you receive from your own health care provider. Together, let's solve your child's and family's food allergy and sensitivity problems.

7

Milk Allergy and Sensitivity

We all grew up hearing the slogan "Milk: it does a body good." This morphed into the more hip catchphrase, "Got milk?" And what is it now? Milk life? These ad campaigns highlight the fact that milk is an integral part of modern nutrition, which holds true in many countries. We know that human babies thrive on human breast milk; this is Mother Nature's nutrition at its very best. We do our best to simulate breast milk with cow's milk–based formulas for those who can't breastfeed, although this simulation isn't nearly as close as it needs to be. We also know that animals thrive on the milk of their own species. All mammals require this high-fat, high-protein, nutrient-rich, and healthy sugar-based food source during the early years of rapid brain and body growth. This milk really is the nutritional basis of all mammalian life on our planet.

But what about beyond infancy and toddlerhood? Do humans really need to drink cow's milk? Does cow's milk do *every* body good? Are humans even supposed to drink the milk of another species? Should we routinely give our kids a glass of milk with every meal, as many American households do? These are interesting questions, and we would argue that the answer is both yes and no. On the yes side, those who are not allergic or sensitive to milk can enjoy it as part of their diet. It provides a healthy source of calcium and protein. Whole milk is an excellent source of fat for toddlers (if weaned from breastfeeding), especially during the years of picky eating. Yogurt and cheese are valuable probiotic-rich foods. Butter, sour cream, ice cream, whipped cream, and cream in our coffee: where would we be without these seemingly essential items? The Sears families have enjoyed milk and milk products for generations, and none of us seem to be sensitive or allergic to it.

However, we believe that there is nothing inherently essential about drinking cow's milk. A toddler can get everything he or she needs nutritionally from eating a well-balanced diet of fruits, vegetables, meat, fish, nuts, eggs, legumes, grains, and any other food that a family typically eats. Cow's milk doesn't have to be part of the human diet—we view it as optional. If a child likes milk, go ahead and let him drink it, and watch for allergy or sensitivity to make sure he is handling it. If a child doesn't like it, there's no reason to push it—just go without. There are plenty of nonmilk sources of calcium, fat, and protein that kids will eat instead.

My kids don't drink milk on a daily basis. We *use* milk for things that require it, such as to put on cereal and to dip our homemade chocolate chip cookies in. Our teens sometimes drink a glass here and there. But we have never made milk an everyday part of our family's diet. We just never needed it, and our kids preferred to drink water.

Surprisingly, though, you will hear doctors, nutritionists, and other medical professionals advise people to drink three glasses of milk every day, as if it's a necessary part of human nutrition that no one should go without. There is no scientific basis for this recommendation. We believe that milk has become ingrained in our society basically through good advertising, not as a result of any research-based findings.

So drink milk if you and your children like it, but don't push it. And when investigating food allergies and sensitivities, cow's milk should be the first thing to go.

WHY MILK MAY *NOT* DO A BODY GOOD

Milk allergy, as we will discuss in the rest of this chapter, is not the only potential problem with cow's milk. What we, as a society, allow to be put into conventional cow's milk is dangerous to our health. We are referring to pesticides, antibiotics, and growth hormones. These three ingredients can cause considerable harm, especially during the formative years of infancy and young childhood. Here are some specific concerns:

Pesticides

Most cows in America are fed conventionally grown grass, grain, and other foods, which contain pesticides, just as our own human food supply does. These pesticides find their way into the cow's milk, onto our dinner tables, and into our children. A 2004 USDA report revealed that 30 percent of nonorganic cow's milk contains measurable levels of pesticides. It is a known fact, confirmed by numerous research studies, that pesticides cause cancer, birth defects, and allergy and neurological disorders. These pesticides are allowed because our society *hopes* that the amount in our diet is too little to cause noticeable harm. We disagree.

Growth Hormones

Cows raised to provide conventional milk are injected with growth hormones to boost milk production. Six types of growth hormones are used. The worst of these are the genetically modified hormones identified by the names rBST and rBGH. They entered the US dairy market in the early 1990s, though they are actually banned in most industrialized countries because of their link to cancer. Numerous reports have been published regarding concerns with these hormones. As a result, many milk farmers in the United States no longer put these particular hormones into their cows. But unfortunately, they are still used to some degree. Look for labels that say *rBST-free* or *rBGH-free*. We should point out, though, that other hormones are used in conventional cow's milk that are not listed on the labels. When buying milk, organic is definitely the safest way to go to avoid growth hormones.

Antibiotics

These are routinely fed to cows, chickens, and other food animals to prevent infection. Unfortunately, trace levels of these drugs then find their way into the milk supply. Studies have found an association between antibiotic exposure and allergic disorders, which is another example of why organic is best.

So if you are a milk-drinking family, we strongly advise that you invest in organic milk. And you have to be vigilant. You have to make sure *all* your milk products are organic: yogurt, cheese, butter, ice cream, everything. It's safe to say that almost nobody is 100 percent organic with all these choices. But be aware that exposing an infant or toddler to these chemicals can contribute to allergic disorders.

HOW TO DIAGNOSE MILK ALLERGY AND SENSITIVITY

Investigating milk allergy and sensitivity is a three-step process: identifying symptoms, testing, and performing elimination trials to observe improvement.

Symptoms Specific to Milk Allergy and Sensitivity

You read about general signs of food allergy and sensitivity in Chapter 6. Here is a recap of the most common signs that apply specifically to milk:

Nasal and respiratory congestion. Chronic symptoms that cannot be attributed to illness or do not vary with seasons of the year are likely to be milk allergy. Asthma can also be a symptom.

Intestinal symptoms. Chronic runny or mucusy stools should be attributed to milk until proven otherwise. Milk is also a common cause of constipation due to a chemical sensitivity to milk proteins.

Recurrent sinus and ear infections. These recurrent infections are a common scenario in toddlers who start milk at age one. Milk allergy can trigger them, and this can then lead to antibiotic overuse. The persistent allergy and antibiotic combination is a double whammy that profoundly affects the health of the intestines and immune system and perpetuates the cycle of recurrent infections.

Rash. Eczema and other chronic rashes can be a sign of milk allergy.

Behavioral reactions. Milk sensitivity can trigger colic in infants, tantrums in toddlers, and defiance or hyperactivity in children.

Testing for Milk Allergy and Sensitivity

You've learned about food allergy testing in Chapter 6. Here are some milk-specific choices:

Milk IgE blood and skin tests. These are very accurate in older children and adults, but they may not show a positive result for infants and toddlers, even when the allergy is present. We routinely do blood IgE food panels for children of any age with persistent classic allergy symptoms (nasal, respiratory, intestinal, or skin). If blood tests don't prove useful, we refer to an allergist for skin testing.

Milk IgE component blood test. If you have a positive skin or blood result to milk, you can get a more accurate breakdown of this allergy with a component blood test, which will determine exactly which milk protein you are allergic to. Three main proteins in milk are involved in allergies: lactalbumin, lactoglobulin, and casein. The first two proteins are heat-sensitive, meaning they break down and lose much of their allergic potential when cooked. Those who are only allergic to lactalbumin and lactoglobulin can usually eat foods with milk ingredients cooked in them and are likely to outgrow this allergy. In fact, about 80 percent of allergic children will outgrow their milk allergy by the teen years. Casein, on the other hand, remains allergenic when cooked and is more likely to create a lifelong allergy or sensitivity. Getting this detailed test can help guide your dietary choices and reintroduction decisions in the coming years.

Milk IgG blood test. This test for milk sensitivity or delayed allergy may help reveal whether milk is a factor in chronic allergic disease, behavioral problems, or developmental delay. It is not accurate in the first year of life, and page 113 discusses the uncertain accuracy of this test in children and adults. We perform this test in some children with chronic problems.

Milk peptide urine test. A small percentage of people do not digest milk properly; some of the poorly digested milk proteins take on a structure that is similar to morphine. This can have a druglike effect. Gluten can cause this same problem, and on page 158 we explain this theory in more depth. These morphine-like milk proteins can be measured in the urine. A high level may be an indication of chemical sensitivity to milk, which can cause intestinal symptoms (especially constipation), behavioral problems, or developmental delay. In our experience, most children with a suspected milk sensitivity will show a positive result on this test. However, we do not often use this test because its accuracy has not been validated by any mainstream medical research. A milk-free trial is more accurate.

Testing for lactose intolerance. Instead of an allergy to milk, those with lactose intolerance lack the intestinal enzyme necessary to digest milk *sugar* (lactose). The undigested sugar ferments into gas within the gut, causing pain, bloating, and diarrhea. Three tests are available. One is a blood test, but it isn't very accurate. A stool acidity analysis is the easiest test to do, particularly in children. But the most accurate one is a hydrogen breath test. Performed in a hospital lab, this test analyzes the exhaled air for elevated hydrogen gas generated by undigested lactose.

Elimination and Observation Trial

Allergy specialists generally agree that the most accurate way to diagnose a food allergy or sensitivity is to witness reactions when the food is eaten, to see the reactions subside when the food is eliminated, and to observe the reactions once again when the food is reintroduced.

Create a food diary chart. Write down the specific symptoms and problems that you attribute to food allergy and sensitivity. Mark the date on your calendar when you first start the diet, and write down your daily observations regarding the symptoms. Don't rely on memory alone; hard data help make the diagnosis more clear.

Elimination trial. Remove all sources of milk, milk products, and milk ingredients from the diet, as outlined below under "Other Milk-Related Foods." Positive results may be seen right away, or several weeks may be required to witness improvements. The timing of results varies among individuals. If you see improvement, you can consider your child (or yourself) allergic or sensitive to milk. Remain completely milk-free for at least three months to allow the immune system to recover and adjust and to let the benefits sink in. Use this time to confirm that improvements are truly sustained.

Rechallenge trial. The decision to reintroduce milk depends on the severity of symptoms and the response to elimination. If the allergy or sensitivity was severe to begin with and the improvements are obvious during milk elimination, you don't need to test the theory with reintroduction. If you are uncertain as to whether or not going off milk has helped, you can reintroduce it to see if symptoms return. This can help solidify the diagnosis one way or the other. Be sure to continue charting your progress in your diary.

Your milk-free diet doesn't have to remain strict forever. Once you have made the diagnosis and have lived milk-free for a few months, you can carefully explore some of the least allergenic milk-based foods to see if you (or your child) can tolerate them. Yogurt, cheese, kefir, and raw milk are tolerated by many people who are milk-sensitive or allergic (see below), and some children will be fine with milk that's cooked into food. Time will tell.

Other Milk-Related Foods

Many foods come from milk: yogurt, cheese, butter, cream, and ice cream are the primary ones. Milk and milk products are also ingredients in most baked foods, like bread, cake, and cookies. Frozen, canned, and dried foods often contain powdered milk or the milk proteins whey and casein. Then there are other animal-based milks, like goat and camel milk. We recommend that you eliminate *all* these sources of milk during the initial months of an elimination trial for the best possible results.

Some people who are milk-sensitive or allergic can tolerate yogurt and cheese fairly well. The fermentation process that these foods undergo reduces their allergic potential. Camel and goat milk are less allergenic and may be tolerated by some cow's milk–allergic people. Some may even tolerate cow's milk baked into recipes. Finally, raw cow's milk may not cause allergic reactions in allergic people, because it is usually well tolerated in its natural form. Trial and error, along with a detailed written food diary, will answer these questions for you.

HOW TO BALANCE A MILK-FREE DIET

For some families, milk is so ingrained in the diet that the very thought of living without it causes chills. Most toddlers are fairly picky eaters, and cow's milk may seem to be the only thing keeping your toddler alive. Snacks and school lunches are often dairy-based, and you don't want your child to feel "different" from the other kids. And what about eating out and enjoying all those dairy-based desserts? Even cream in your coffee is hard to imagine living without. Nobody wants to go milk-free unless they have to. But if you and your doctor have determined that someone in your family is milk-allergic or milk-sensitive, you will need to adopt a milk-free diet. Here's a bit of good news, though: as you just read, some people are sensitive only to straight milk and can tolerate many other forms of milk-based foods. So the toughest time will be during the initial elimination trial, when you will avoid all sources of milk. Then you can ease in some of the least allergenic forms of milk, like yogurt and cheese, and see how they are tolerated (see info below).

Here are instructions (listed according to the age of your child) for safely eliminating milk and milk products without compromising your family's nutrition and cramping your lifestyle:

Infants Younger than Age One

If you are a breastfeeding mom, you will eliminate all sources of cow's milk from your diet, and you won't give your baby any milk-based foods when starting solids. It may take a couple of weeks to see your infant improve as the milk proteins leave your body and your milk. Follow the instructions below ("Older Infants and Children") to help make sure your diet is complete. Do not give up breastfeeding; your baby is already getting off to a rough start in life having to deal with allergies and sensitivities. Ongoing breast milk (with the allergens eliminated) is a crucial element in your baby's overall nutritional and immune health, and it will greatly lower the risk of further allergic disorders. Switching to formula may provide short-term relief from allergies passing through your milk, but not without the long-term consequences of losing all the benefits of extended breastfeeding.

If you are not breastfeeding and are instead using a milk-based formula, discuss the various formula options with your doctor. In our experience, milk-allergic infants tolerate the following formulas, listed in order of preference (the least allergenic and most nutritious listed first):

Donated breast milk. Breast milk is always going to be the most nutritious choice for an infant. If you cannot supply your own breast milk, seek donations from trusted family members or friends, or obtain a supply from a milk bank. Even if the milk donors are not cow's milk–free themselves, this breast milk may be better tolerated than formula.

Homemade infant formula with raw milk or goat milk. Because raw milk is considerably less allergenic than the pasteurized, homogenized milk used in formula, this may be a good option for your baby if approved by your physician. Various recipes are available online for those who want to make it themselves, and some home-based businesses sell batches of homemade formula. Organic ingredients should include raw whole milk, cream, various oils (flax, cod liver, coconut, olive, or sunflower), nutritional yeast (a good source of many vitamins and minerals), gelatin (for digestion), extra lactose, water, and probiotics. Goat milk (usually not available raw) can be used in place of cow's milk, as the proteins are less allergenic and more easily digested. Warning: such formulas are neither FDA regulated nor approved, and you should use one only with the guidance and approval of your physician.

Low-lactose or lactose-free formula. These formulas are available for infants who are lactose intolerant (meaning they cannot fully digest milk sugar). Testing for this condition usually isn't done, but a successful trial with the formula can make the diagnosis. As an alternative, lactase digestive enzyme drops (available OTC) can be added to a milk-based formula to aid in lactose digestion.

Hypoallergenic infant formula. Various specialized formulas are available for milk-allergic infants. Some contain milk protein but may be well tolerated. Your doctor will guide you through these choices.

Soy formula. This is not a good option, as some who are allergic to milk will also be allergic to soy. Also, soy is not a complete protein, and there are some medical concerns about using soy as a primary nutritional source during infancy. This should be a last resort.

Older Infants and Children

If your toddler has been dairy-free growing up, she won't know what she's missing, and remaining dairy-free will be fairly easy. This is not necessarily so for the toddler who is already hooked on milk and cheese. Removing these products from the diet can bring out the most persistent protests, so be ready. Older kids, who have more verbal skills and with whom you can reason, generally accept the idea that they are allergic to milk and should comply with the changes, especially if they feel better on the diet. Here are guidelines for a healthy dairy-free diet for children:

Alternative milk source. Continue breastfeeding as long as mutually desired by baby and Mom. No other source of milk is needed. If using formula, continue this into the second year of life as long as you and your doctor think it's appropriate. Once your child is weaned, an alternative milk source isn't necessarily needed, but it may be desired for comfort routines, for use on cereal or in smoothies, or with anything else for which you need "milk." Here are some calcium-enriched choices instead of milk, in order of nutritional preference:

- Hemp milk, made from hemp seeds, has one of the highest protein contents of all the alternative milks, along with a healthy amount of fat and carbs.
- Coconut milk has the highest fat content, which is useful for toddlers, but it has very little protein or carbs.
- Almond, rice, and potato milks are mostly carbs, with very little fat or protein.
- Soy milk is the closest nutritional match to cow's milk (same amount of fat, only slightly less protein, and fewer carbs), but it has too much allergic potential in those who are allergic to milk. We don't recommend using it regularly.

- Use unsweetened milks as much as possible. The sugar content of sweetened alternative milks is generally too high.
- Goat milk. Some people who are allergic to cow's milk are also allergic to goat milk. However, goat milk is significantly less allergenic than cow's milk; we routinely advise our milk-allergic patients to try goat milk and see if it's tolerated. And if your reaction to milk involves only digestive problems, you may find goat milk easier on the stomach.
- Nondairy milk products are also available: cheese, yogurt, and butter made from nonmilk sources can replace these favorite foods.

It may be best to mix and match these milks — for example, a combination of hemp and coconut milks will provide the most protein and fat. Alternate among the various types to vary your child's nutrition and tastes.

Calcium source. Whenever someone goes milk-free, the first worry that enters the mind is calcium. During the initial months of a dairy-free diet, don't panic if your child won't increase other calcium sources right away. Young bodies have plenty of stored calcium to see a child through at least several months. Once you've been dairy-free for about three months and are seeing the benefits, you can start introducing yogurt, cheese, and kefir, which provide everything milk does. If your child does well with these items, you've found your calcium source. If you determine that these cause allergy or sensitivity symptoms, you'll have to begin nondairy sources of calcium. The alternative milks above have the same amount of calcium as regular milk, which equals about 30 percent of the daily requirement per eight-ounce cup. Here are some other ideas, along with their approximate calcium content per serving:

- Sardines (3 ounces) — 371 milligrams
- Calcium-fortified orange juice (1 cup) — 300 milligrams

- Chickpeas (1 cup)—300 milligrams
- Sesame seeds (1 ounce)—280 milligrams
- Spinach (1 cup)—272 milligrams (although calcium in spinach isn't well absorbed due to its oxalate content)
- Kale and collard greens (1 cup)—179 to 357 milligrams
- Tofu (organic, non-GMO, 3 ounces)—190 milligrams
- Broccoli (1 cup)—177 milligrams
- Rhubarb (½ cup)—174 milligrams
- Salmon (canned, 3 ounces)—167 milligrams
- Refried beans (1 cup)—141 milligrams
- Blackstrap molasses (1 tablespoon)—137 milligrams
- Artichoke (1 medium)—135 milligrams
- Figs (5)—135 milligrams
- Almond butter (2 tablespoons)—86 milligrams
- Dried apricots (1 cup)—59 milligrams
- Dried beans (cooked, 1 cup)—50 to 100 milligrams

Toddlers and children need about 800 milligrams of dietary calcium every day. Teens need about twice that amount. If necessary, you can supplement with calcium in liquid, chewable, or tablet form under your doctor's direction.

Protein and fat. Milk and milk products are convenient sources of protein and fat, especially during the toddler years when children most need these nutrients and won't eat a wide variety of foods. Here are the healthiest foods you can give your toddler that replace the necessary fat and protein content of milk:

- Fish (especially wild salmon)
- Lean meat (skinless poultry, wild game, grass-fed beef)
- Eggs
- Nuts and nut butters (and seeds and seed butters)
- Oils (flax, olive, coconut)

- Avocados
- Legumes
- Whole grains

General cooking and baking. Some milk-allergic people find they can tolerate milk as an ingredient in baked foods. For those who can't, countless recipe books and websites provide plenty of suggestions on how to cook and bake dairy-free. Here are a few ideas on what you can substitute for commonly used dairy products in your kitchen:

- Milk can be replaced one for one with any of the alternative milks listed above, or even with water or fruit juice.
- Yogurt can be replaced with equal portions of soy or coconut yogurt, soy sour cream, unsweetened applesauce, or fruit puree.
- Butter has plenty of alternatives: margarine, oil-based spreads, shortening (not very healthy), or oils (coconut, olive, or vegetable).
- Even evaporated milk has some options: use canned coconut milk, or evaporate some of the water out of rice or almond milk by gently boiling it down to half the volume.
- Buttermilk: add 1 tablespoon of lemon juice or white vinegar to your substitute milk and let it stand until thick.

Treats. Let's be realistic: Kids need treats. So do adults. Going dairy-free eliminates some of the yummiest desserts, like ice cream and many baked recipes. Here are some ideas that will help satisfy the sweet tooth in all of us:

- Nondairy ice cream (rice, coconut, or other types)
- Dark chocolate treats (instead of milk chocolate)
- 100 percent frozen-juice pops

- Google *dairy-free desserts for kids* and you'll see all kinds of choices, from cookies and brownies to caramel popcorn and peanut brittle. Even dark chocolate peanut butter cups are a hit.

HOW LONG CAN A TODDLER GO WITHOUT EATING?

When you first eliminate milk, your toddler may protest with a hunger strike. Your most creative attempts to offer food may be met with closed lips and a turned head. It's difficult for a parent to watch her child go days without much nutrition; it goes against all your parental instincts. But hang in there! No child will allow himself to remain malnourished to an extent that causes harm. The one exception to this is children with developmental delays who have extreme oral aversions; the resistance in such kids may be a tough nut to crack. With most kids, however, hunger will kick in and food will eventually be consumed. And don't push the food too hard; many toddlers will resist simply because they sense you want them to eat. You yourself should prepare food, sit down and eat three meals a day, and keep snacks at hand for your enjoyment. Let your child watch you without any prompting or pressure. If you're not trying to coax him into eating, he may feel that you don't want him to eat—in which case he will likely try to do the opposite and actually start eating, just to show you who's in charge. Once your toddler discovers this self-motivation to eat, you can move on and watch for improvements on the milk-free diet.

REINTRODUCING MILK PRODUCTS: TESTING YOUR TOLERANCE AND ROTATING YOUR DIET

You've eliminated milk and milk products for a few months and observed the alleviation of your child's allergy or sensitivity symptoms, but now the kids are whining for some of their old favorite foods. Can you safely reintroduce milk products? Possibly. This depends on several factors. If your child's difficulties with milk were severe, and the changes in health or behavior were dramatic, we recommend that you commit to being completely milk-free and milk product–free for as many years as you can. The immune system will likely remember this severe allergy for several years at least, and other body systems may remain sensitive for a while as well. Let your child enjoy a healthy and happy early childhood, unencumbered by immune, gastrointestinal, allergic, and behavioral problems. This is particularly important during the first five years of life, when the immune and neurological systems are growing and developing rapidly. You can gradually reintroduce products later, with your doctor's guidance.

If your child's milk allergies or sensitivities were mild, you can safely and carefully reintroduce some milk products after just a few months. Your child's body will need less time to heal with a mild allergy than a severe one, and the immune system may have lost some of its allergic memory by this point. Your child is likely to tolerate some milk products, as long as you don't overdo it.

For those with moderate milk problems who lie somewhere in between, you and your doctor should decide how long to remain milk-free. When you do feel ready, this section will guide you through the process.

Repeating Allergy Tests

If your or your child's difficulties were primarily allergic in nature and you had positive allergic results during your initial tests, it's useful to repeat the testing before reintroducing any milk products. Your allergy specialist will counsel you on this step. This is particularly important for those with a history of severe allergy. If the allergy was mild to moderate, repeat testing isn't absolutely necessary. Remember, the most accurate laboratory is the human body. An allergist may advise reintroducing foods without testing first, instead using observation as your guide.

For those with milk *sensitivities*, repeating any tests is not necessary. Remember, the reliability of milk sensitivity testing (IgG food antibodies, urine peptide tests) isn't certain to begin with. Some people with positive test results will go on to show normal results after being on a restricted diet. But research has not yet been done to corroborate that this finding really means the sensitivity is gone. Repeat testing for sensitivities is not worth the time and money, in our opinion.

Safest Foods with Which to Start

Don't just hand your child a glass of milk and say "Enjoy!" Here are the least allergenic forms of milk, listed in the order in which they should be reintroduced:

Yogurt. Yogurt is made by fermenting milk with healthy bacteria and yeast, and many kids can tolerate it again without allergic or sensitive reactions. Use organic brands.

Raw milk. Raw milk is much less allergenic than conventional milk and is easily tolerated by many sensitive people. Review the box below for more information.

Ghee and butter. These milk derivatives contain little to no milk proteins, so they will likely be tolerated.

Cheese. Cheese is also made by a fermentation process, and the healthy mold and bacteria in cheese may help reduce its allergic potential. The harder the cheese, the less likely it is to trigger allergic reactions in some people (because hard cheeses have less whey protein and more casein protein).

Kefir. This liquid yogurt drink is also made by fermentation. Some will tolerate it well, especially those with lactose intolerance, as most of its lactose sugar is consumed in the fermentation process.

Milk as an ingredient in foods. Try some baked goods or packaged foods with milk as a minor ingredient. If these are tolerated, try some favorite milk-based foods, like ice cream and pizza (you're really going wild now!).

Milk (finally!). Save the real milk for last, and definitely make the switch to organic milk. Start slowly, with half a glass at a time.

RAW MILK: OKAY FOR MILK-SENSITIVE PEOPLE?

Smart pediatricians learn from their patients, and we've observed a surprising phenomenon in our practice: some children who are sensitive or allergic to conventional cow's milk can tolerate raw cow's milk without any noticeable symptoms. We don't happen to drink raw milk in our family, and we doctors are taught that raw milk is dangerous. Raw milk can be contaminated with infectious bacteria that cause severe food poisoning when unsanitary practices are followed at a dairy farm. So until recently, we had never recommended it to patients. But some progressive moms in our office have put their families on raw, organic cow's milk, and we've seen their allergic or sensitive children do just fine. Why is this so? Conventional milk goes through heat pasteurization to kill bacteria. The problem is that this kills all the live properties in milk: the antibodies, healthy probiotic bacteria, enzymes, growth factors, and other nutrients. Heat also alters the milk proteins. Furthermore, the homogenization process that binds all the proteins, fats, and sugars together so they

(continued)

don't separate presents the final milk product to us in an altered form that may not be intended for human consumption. Milk is supposed to separate easily for digestion.

Conventional milk is certainly safer from an infectious disease viewpoint, but its altered chemistry and biology may be a large reason why so many people have allergic or digestive reactions to it. We believe that raw milk is a better, healthier way to go, and that it can be a safe alternative for families who are sensitive or allergic. You can virtually eliminate the risk of food poisoning by carefully researching your local raw milk dairy farm's history and practices; a farm with a good track record is a safe choice.

How Much, How Often

You have to be careful to introduce these foods gradually. Begin with about half of a serving (serving size listed on the label) once. Watch how your child does over the course of that week. If all is well, continue that food once a week for a month. If no reactions develop, allow a full serving once each week. Add a second food type a few days apart from the first (a full-sized serving is fine), and continue that new food once each week. For example, give yogurt every Monday and a food with cheese in it every Thursday. As long as your child is doing well, continue this process. Throw in some milk-containing foods on a different day of the week. Work up to feeding your child one of these foods every day and shorten the intervals between servings of the same food—for example, enjoying cheese every four days instead of every seven. But stay away from straight milk during this process, as it is the most allergic of these foods. Try using raw milk if you like. If you detect problems along the way with a particular type of milk product, stop that particular food, back off all milk products for a few weeks, and then resume without that food.

You'll learn what is tolerated and what is not, and with what frequency each product can be consumed.

This concept of feeding a food about every four to seven days is called a rotation diet. It allows a person to enjoy the food without overloading the immune and intestinal system too frequently. If you continually encounter problems as you increase the dairy, you may find that you have to restrict all dairy foods to once every four to seven days. Enjoy yogurt one day, then a meal with cheese five days later, followed by a frozen yogurt treat four days after that. If reactions continue to occur, you may need to commit to being completely dairy-free for the long term.

IS THERE SOME MILK AT THE END OF THE TUNNEL?

Want your child to outgrow his milk allergy? Want to enjoy dairy again yourself? Some are lucky enough to have this happen automatically. We observe that most of our patients outgrow their milk allergy or sensitivity as they progress through childhood. Many sensitive toddlers go on to eat a regular diet by the time they hit kindergarten. Some lose their allergy at an older age. This is a very unpredictable process, but studies show that about 75 percent of children will outgrow their milk allergy by the time they are teenagers.

Some will have to work at it, though. Oral desensitization therapy for milk allergy is being investigated and shows promising results so far. Under the guidance of an allergist, gradually increasing amounts of milk protein are consumed over a period of time. Some people will learn to tolerate it without significant reactions. If approved, this treatment will provide relief for those who don't outgrow their milk allergy.

Until then, there are many things you can do to help decrease your allergic reactivity, heal the gut, and improve your neurological health—which may improve the odds that you'll outgrow a milk allergy (and *all* food allergies, for that matter). In Chapter 14, we teach you how to eat properly to reduce inflammation and improve immune health. We show you how to improve intestinal health and guard your gut against inflammatory insults. After your child has lived for a few years without dairy products irritating the gut and stimulating the allergic side of the immune system, and when you and your family make the right nutritional, lifestyle, and health care choices, your child's body may be able to handle these foods once again. The immune system never completely loses its memory of this allergy, but with a healthier gut and immune system, the reaction may be minimal. Embrace Chapter 14; it will be your family's ticket to wellness.

8

Wheat and Gluten Allergy and Sensitivity

You've just made it through the milk allergy chapter. If your head is already spinning, you'd better sit down to read this next chapter. What we have to share with you regarding wheat and gluten allergy and sensitivity is both profound and controversial: profound because the harmful effects gluten can have on a sensitive body are shocking and far-reaching, and controversial because some doctors don't yet believe that gluten sensitivity is a real entity.

Gluten is one of several proteins in wheat. It is responsible for making wheat dough stretchy and helps it to rise. Gluten is also a component of several other grains, including barley and rye. As you will read below, gluten is the component of wheat that is most often responsible for wheat sensitivity—though there are other proteins in wheat that can also trigger allergic reactions, independent of gluten.

We Sears doctors have helped pave various inroads into modern parenting practices and children's health care. Dr. Bill was among the first American doctors to promote long-term breast-feeding, and now everybody's doing it. He was also among the first to tell parents it's okay to co-sleep with your baby, especially if it gives the family a good night's rest. And he started the movement of attachment parenting. Who knew that bonding with babies could be so beneficial? I have entered the ring by providing alternative approaches to childhood vaccination as a way to help keep vaccination rates high, and I have offered insights into alternative nutritional and medical treatments for autism and other developmental delays. Gluten sensitivity is our latest project because it's real, it's harmful, it's largely unrecognized, and it's affecting members of our own family.

I went gluten-free about nine months before beginning this book. The prompt for that change came when two members of my family were diagnosed with autoimmune thyroid disease. Our endocrinologist advised them to go gluten-free to help calm down their immune systems. I decided to join them in their experiment without even retesting myself (I'd had normal wheat and gluten test results several years ago). I was pleasantly surprised to see my asthma virtually disappear. I've advised numerous allergic patients to go gluten-free but had never thought to try it for my own asthma.

Some have said that going gluten-free is just a fad. One patient said those very words as I displayed her child's positive gluten sensitivity test results and explained why he was having chronic medical problems. But it's not a fad. Numerous mainstream research papers have been published by gastroenterology and allergy specialists worldwide, describing this newly recognized disorder, which has been termed non-celiac gluten sensitivity. We will just call it gluten sensitivity for short.

So why the controversy, and why are many doctors skeptical about this disorder? We believe two factors are involved: the fact that virtually none of the doctors currently in medical practice have received training in non-celiac gluten sensitivity, and the confusion created by patients who insisted they had celiac disease (a severe autoimmune disorder) when, in fact, they only had non-celiac gluten sensitivity.

This first factor can be easily remedied by participating in continuing medical education seminars or keeping up to date with mainstream medical journals. But many doctors don't have the time for these, and when they do make the time, they focus their studies on the areas that interest them the most. Many won't yet have read or learned about gluten sensitivity. So when they're presented with it in their office, it doesn't exist to them. And when patients ask about it, these doctors dismiss their worries and advise them to stop reading Google.

The second factor is probably the primary contributor to the controversy. In the 1990s, when people started worrying about gluten causing anything from stomachaches to chronic fatigue, many thought they had celiac disease, a severe autoimmune disorder in which the immune system reacts so strongly to gluten that it attacks many other organs in the body, particularly the GI system and the brain. Those with unrecognized celiac disease often have chronic and severe diarrhea, poor growth, weight loss, and sometimes neuropsychiatric symptoms. Many people went to their doctors with their worries, and the doctors pooh-poohed their concerns because these patients didn't seem sick enough to have true celiac disease. And the doctors were right— this wasn't true celiac disease. But no one knew about non-celiac gluten sensitivity. So the rising incidence of gluten sensitivity was largely ignored by the medical community, and in fact it still is today. But one by one, doctors are coming around as more and more research is being published about the disorder.

The bottom line on gluten and wheat is that they can be responsible for a myriad of health problems. True celiac disease is fairly rare, but gluten sensitivity is not. This chapter will guide you through the process of determining whether or not your family is sensitive and what you should do about it.

WHY WHEAT AND GLUTEN SENSITIVITY IS SO COMMON TODAY

A growing number of doctors and researchers are now blowing the whistle on wheat and gluten. Two particularly well-written books on this subject are *Grain Brain* by neurologist Dr. David Perlmutter and *Wheat Belly* by cardiologist Dr. William Davis. These are good reads and valuable tools for those who are looking to lose weight, improve their heart and brain health, and reduce symptoms of chronic disease. They also shed some light on how our nation's wheat has changed over the past fifty years to cause so much sensitivity.

The wheat we eat today is very different than what our ancestors ate. In its original form, wheat is very healthy and has been a staple of the diet worldwide. The problem comes from what we've done to it in the past half century. Agricultural scientists have hybridized and crossbred wheat to make it more resistant to drought and fungi and to increase the yield of wheat crops. The genetic makeup of modern wheat is very different from ancient wheat. One species of ancient wheat has fourteen chromosomes in its genetic code. Another has twenty-eight. Today's manipulated wheat has forty-two chromosomes, and the genes that regulate gluten production and function are a particular target of these genetic alterations. Modern wheat has more gluten proteins than ancient wheat, and the number and structure of the various other proteins in wheat has also changed (specifically, today's gluten has been bred to make it easier to bake with).

The result is that our digestive and immune systems now react to wheat in a very different way; we treat wheat and gluten as foreign invaders, not as nutrients. Some published studies propose that celiac disease and gluten sensitivity are caused by these genetic changes in wheat and gluten. Drs. Davis and Perlmutter offer numerous research references in their books to back up their theories, and provide information on how ancient strains of wheat can safely be enjoyed as part of a healthy diet. The two most popular ancient strains are einkorn and emmer, which are available from some local farms and numerous online retailers.

Technically, today's wheat is not actually genetically modified, like corn and soy. Nothing artificial has been inserted into its genes. So modern wheat can be labeled "non-GMO," which gives people the false impression that it is healthy and natural. Another factor that has made wheat particularly harmful is that it has become so prevalent in the American diet; it's in every meal, and in large quantities. Think about it: we all eat wheat for breakfast (cereal, pancakes, waffles, toast, bagels, doughnuts), wheat for lunch (bread), wheat for snacks (crackers, pretzels, bars), wheat for dinner (breaded foods, pasta, bread again), and wheat for dessert (cake, cookies, pie). As a species, we were designed to enjoy some ancient wheat—but to do so in moderation, as we also consume meat, fish, vegetables, fruits, nuts, seeds, and healthy oils. Perhaps the *quantity* of wheat is the primary concern, not the *quality*.

In this chapter you will learn how to determine whether you have gluten sensitivity, wheat allergy, or full-blown celiac disease, and what you can do about it. We will also tell you how even those who aren't sensitive can benefit from reducing wheat consumption.

NEGATIVE METABOLIC EFFECTS OF WHEAT AND GLUTEN: BEYOND ALLERGIES

Wheat allergy isn't the only problem. Eating too much wheat raises blood sugar and insulin levels, creates more body fat, contributes to bad cholesterol, and triggers autoimmune reactions throughout the body. Wheat and gluten can negatively affect *all* of us, not just those who are sensitive or allergic. Here is how:

(continued)

Elevated Blood Sugar and Insulin: The Beginning of Diabetes

Modern whole wheat has a high glycemic index, almost as high as table sugar and white bread. The digestive process basically turns wheat into sugar, causing a particularly high blood sugar level, an insulin rush, followed by a sugar low. We are basically pouring sugar down our throats with every meal and snack. This wear and tear on the pancreas (the organ that generates insulin in response to sugar) contributes to a higher risk of diabetes. Studies have shown that children with insulin-dependent diabetes are more likely to have a positive gluten sensitivity test result, and have up to a twenty-fold higher chance of developing celiac disease.

If and when diabetes finally takes its hold on the body, sugar begins depositing itself in various body tissues, alters the protein structure, and causes gradual degeneration, particularly in the joints, eyes, kidneys, blood vessels, and brain.

This sugar phenomenon isn't unique to wheat, however. Many grains cause a similar swing in blood sugar and insulin. In Chapter 14, you'll read more about the benefit of reducing all grains in the diet.

Visceral Fat: Slow-Acting Poison That Wreaks Havoc on the Body

Any extra sugar or carb that is consumed in a meal and not readily used by the body for energy is stored as fat. Much of this fat is healthy and is readily broken down again for energy when the body needs it. However, wheat carbs have a particular tendency to be stored as visceral fat, the fat in our belly. This fat is not easily burned away. But even worse, visceral fat continuously secretes inflammatory molecules. In Chapter 1, you learned how the immune system releases inflammatory molecules in response to illness, injury, and infection. These molecules help the body rid itself of foreign invaders and help us heal. But inflammation is also destructive. Imagine these harmful molecules leaking continuously into the bloodstream unchecked. This chronic inflammatory wear and tear from visceral fat damages the heart, blood vessels, joints, and other body tissues.

Bad Cholesterol: Not Just Caused by Eating Fat

High blood sugar increases production of VLDL cholesterol (the bad type of cholesterol). This deposits itself on the arteries as plaque. Several decades of plaque buildup eventually result in a heart attack or a stroke. This means that a low-fat, low-cholesterol diet isn't enough: a diet low in carbs, especially low in wheat, is also an important part of healthy eating.

Weak Bones: Acidic Properties of Wheat

Wheat is an acid, as are various other foods we eat, like meat. Fruits and vegetables are alkaline, so they balance the acids in our diet. But if we eat too much acid, the bones release calcium to neutralize it. This can result in weak bones and joints. Ever wonder why overweight elderly people need hip replacements? It's not just the wear and tear of the extra weight; it's a combination of the inflammation from visceral fat and the loss of calcium from the bones.

As you can see, overconsumption of wheat will have a profoundly negative effect on all of us, whether or not we have a wheat sensitivity. That's why it's important to realize that everyone can benefit from a low-wheat diet.

HOW TO DIAGNOSE WHEAT ALLERGY AND NON-CELIAC GLUTEN SENSITIVITY

There are three distinct conditions involving wheat and gluten. Wheat allergy describes an IgE-mediated allergic reaction to wheat, which triggers classic allergic symptoms. Gluten sensitivity (officially called non-celiac gluten sensitivity, as noted earlier) describes non-IgE immune, intestinal, and neurological reactions specific to the gluten component of wheat. Celiac disease (CD) is an autoimmune reaction to gluten and is the most severe form of gluten sensitivity. Investigating wheat and gluten problems follows a process similar to the investigation of any other food allergy and sensitivity: identifying symptoms, testing, and elimination trials to observe improvement.

Symptoms Specific to Wheat and Gluten Allergy and Sensitivity

Wheat and gluten tend to primarily cause skin and intestinal allergies, as well as neurological and behavioral reactions, and are less known for causing nasal allergies.

Intestinal symptoms. Wheat can irritate the gut just like milk, causing gas, pain, bloating, diarrhea, and other gut symptoms. These can occur either from direct allergic irritation of the gut or through a mechanism called leaky gut, described in the box on page 158. When you are faced with chronic intestinal symptoms, it's an even bet between milk and wheat. In some cases, it will be both. The chemical effects of gluten may cause constipation in some people (see "Craving and addiction" below).

Rash. Wheat and gluten can trigger the same generic types of allergic rashes (listed on page 109) as other food allergens. Some skin conditions may be a specific indication of gluten sensitivity, but these rashes have other causes as well; gluten can be either a major component or a minor one:

- Keratosis pilaris. This common skin condition can be a sign of wheat allergy. Affecting about 25 percent of Americans, it appears as fine pimples that cover the upper arms and upper legs. Some will have it on the face and back as well.
- Eczema. This chronic skin allergy can be triggered by various foods, and wheat should be considered in every case (see page 94).

- Dermatitis herpetiformis. This rash mimics herpes or shingles outbreaks on the skin but is caused by gluten allergy instead of a virus. It appears as large clusters of small to medium-sized blisters that are extremely itchy.
- Acne. The inflammatory effects of carb overload contribute to acne.
- Recurrent sores on the corners of the mouth or inside the mouth.
- Psoriasis. This disease mimics eczema but is an autoimmune condition that can be caused by gluten sensitivity.
- Vitiligo. Another autoimmune condition, vitiligo is white patches on the skin due to loss of skin pigment.
- Acanthosis nigricans. A condition commonly seen in diabetics, this dark, velvety skin can develop on the back of the neck and in the armpits.
- Other chronic skin conditions. Any type of autoimmune inflammatory skin condition that doesn't respond to conventional treatment could improve with gluten removal.

Behavioral and neurological reactions. The chemical and immune effects of gluten can reach the brain and trigger chronic behavioral, neurological, and even psychiatric symptoms. These behaviors aren't generally immediate and obvious, as are the few hours of hyperactivity that may be seen shortly after ingesting food coloring. Rather, they become a chronic, daily feature of a person's mood, behavior, and overall functioning.

- Infants can suffer from colic and poor sleep.
- Toddlers can show hyperactivity, severe tantrums, and developmental delay (even autism).
- Children may develop difficulty with focus, learning disorders, defiance, behavioral meltdowns, and obsessive-compulsive disorder (OCD).

- Teens and adults report chronic fatigue, difficulty concentrating, problems with balance and coordination, poor muscle control and numbness, and even psychotic behavior.

Asthma. As in my case, wheat and gluten allergy can be a significant factor in asthma.

Craving and addiction. A recently discovered feature of gluten sensitivity is gluten's addictive properties. Several research studies have found that some of us don't digest modern wheat properly due to a lack of the digestive enzyme dipeptidyl peptidase IV, or DPP IV. Some of the resulting gluten protein fragments in our digestive tract very closely resemble the drug morphine. Called gluteomorphin, this protein exerts a morphine-like effect on our brain, resulting in a mild euphoria that makes us crave gluten even more. Stay away from gluten for too long, and some will experience withdrawal symptoms like irritability, anxiety, and aggression. And just as with drugs, chronic use can suppress neurological function, resulting in fatigue, lack of focus, memory problems, and even psychiatric symptoms. Gluteomorphins in the gut may also slow down gut motility and cause constipation. Milk can exert a similar effect with a protein called casomorphin. These "morphin" levels can be measured with a urine test (see page 132), but the accuracy and usefulness of this test is still uncertain.

LEAKY GUT AND ZONULIN

An emerging theory in medicine that may partly explain the rise in food allergies refers to the "leaky gut," introduced on page 24. Gluten can be a trigger for a leaky gut. Here's how:

Intestinal cells regulate the "leakiness" of the intestinal lining by releasing a protein called *zonulin,* which loosens the bond between intestinal cells, creating a space between them through which anything can "leak." In some circumstances this is a good thing; certain intestinal infections cause the gut to temporarily release zonulin, allowing body fluids to enter the gut in order to flush out the infection (diarrhea). Unfortunately, gluten proteins can also trigger the release of zonulin, causing the gaps between intestinal cells to stay open. This leaky gut has three unwanted consequences:

Gluten sensitization. If you suffer from leaky gut, the immune system is hit with a double whammy. First, modern wheat is higher in gluten, so the amount of gluten that is presented to the immune system with each meal is much greater than what nature intended. Second, these gluten proteins have been altered by science, and these unnatural glutens are even more irritating to the immune system. The T lymphocytes are activated, a chronic inflammatory response against gluten begins, and it doesn't end unless gluten is removed.

Other chemicals and toxins. Chemicals and toxins in food that normally should pass out with the stools are instead allowed into the bloodstream through the leaky spaces between cells. These toxins have negative effects on the body and brain.

Multiple food sensitivities. Gluten isn't the only protein to pass through the leaky spaces; many other incompletely digested food proteins will pass into the bloodstream. The immune system views some of these as foreign, because they haven't been properly digested and processed by the intestinal cells. A person may therefore become sensitive or allergic to many foods which the body otherwise wouldn't have been sensitive to.

Fixing a leaky gut is an important step in healing body inflammation, multiple food allergies and sensitivities, and other allergic disorders. In Chapter 14, we explore how to achieve this.

Testing for Wheat and Gluten Allergy and Sensitivity

Chapter 6 introduced you to food allergy testing. Evaluating allergy and sensitivity to wheat and gluten involves the following:

Wheat IgE blood and skin tests. As you read about with milk on page 132, these tests determine whether a person is allergic to wheat. They are more accurate in older children and adults.

Standard wheat and gluten IgG blood test. This test is somewhat controversial, as its accuracy as an indicator of sensitivity has not yet been verified by medical policy makers. As you read on page 23, standard IgG levels can be measured for many foods, wheat and gluten included. Some doctors believe that healthy people should *not* generate IgG antibodies against food, and that the presence of such antibodies to wheat or gluten indicates a problem. However, most people who are tested for these standard antibodies will have some. Does this mean that most people *do* have a problem with gluten, or is the test just too sensitive? The results are given as a number, so perhaps the higher the number, the greater the gluten sensitivity. We don't yet know, because no one has compared lab data to real-life patient experiences to determine how these levels correlate to patient symptoms. We do perform IgG food testing in our practice, but we understand that the results must be interpreted in light of each patient's symptoms and observable reactions to foods. As stated previously, if you are going to test for wheat and gluten IgG sensitivity, you should do so before eliminating the foods from the diet.

Specialized gluten IgG antibody blood tests. Some components of gluten and gluten metabolism can be tested to evaluate for sensitivity (must be done prior to eliminating gluten to be valid). These are accepted as legitimate indicators of sensitivity by mainstream doctors. The only challenge is that they are only abnormal in cases of moderate to severe sensitivity. Those with mild non-celiac gluten sensitivity will usually show normal results with these tests. Therefore, many cases will be missed. We perform these tests in our office, and when they are abnormal they are a clear indication of sensitivity. These tests include:

- Native gliadin IgG antibody level—Gliadin is one of the proteins that make up gluten, and it is thought to be the most specific indicator of sensitivity. A variation of this test, called a *deamidated* gliadin IgA and IgG antibody level, is a newer version that is more specific for celiac disease (severe gluten allergy) and is discussed on page 168. Those who have only non-celiac gluten sensitivity won't register a positive deamidated antibody. The older version, called a *native* gliadin IgG antibody level, is more appropriate for gluten sensitivity testing. Yet most regular labs now run only the deamidated version. Check with your lab before running this test and, if needed, seek out a specialty lab that offers the native version.
- Tissue transglutaminase IgG antibody level (tTG)—The intestinal enzyme transglutaminase is involved in digestion of gluten, but only those with severe sensitivity will create antibodies against it.
- Reticulin IgG antibody level—Reticulin is a fibrous tissue within the intestines, and those with severe gluten sensitivity will create antibodies against it.

Gluten urine peptide test. The gluteomorphin protein described on page 158, which exerts a negative effect on the brain and the gut, can be measured in the urine. In our experience, however, this test is usually normal, even in those whom we later determine to be gluten-sensitive. We rarely use this test.

Gluten antibody saliva and stool tests. Several private laboratories offer these methods of measuring antibodies to gluten. These samples are easier to collect, since they don't involve blood testing. However, the accuracy of the results has not been verified by the FDA or any independent source. We don't yet perform these tests in our office and are waiting for more research before we do.

Observation: the most accurate gluten test. Most researchers and doctors who focus on non-celiac gluten sensitivity agree that the most accurate way to make the diagnosis is to eliminate gluten and observe the response. Enough research just hasn't been done yet to prove the validity of standard IgG antibody testing, and the specialized gluten IgG tests are rarely abnormal.

Our Approach to Gluten Testing

On page 109 we presented the symptoms of food allergy and sensitivity. Gluten and cow's milk are the two most common causes of these problems. Our personal practice with managing gluten sensitivity is still evolving. We see a significant number of infants and children, as well as parents, who we suspect are gluten-sensitive. We know that the most accurate way to proceed is with a trial of gluten elimination, and some parents agree to give it a try. However, many parents are reluctant. Gluten is such a large part of the American diet, and picky eaters pretty much only eat gluten and dairy foods. Good parents don't want their children to waste away, and the fear that a child won't eat anything else prevents many gluten-free trials in our practice.

So we routinely test such children for food allergy and sensitivity and interpret the results accordingly. The tests we most commonly perform are as follows: food IgE antibodies, including wheat; IgG antibodies to wheat, gluten, and milk; IgG panels that measure several dozen foods in some cases; and IgG and

IgA antibodies to gliadin and tTG (see page 160). We like to run a native gliadin IgG test as well, but this is only offered by some specialty labs and may not be covered by insurance. We don't do saliva and stool tests, and we rarely do the urine test. Blood tests are our standard of care. If the IgE antibody test is positive, the choice to eliminate wheat is easy. If many of the wheat, gluten, or gliadin IgG tests are highly abnormal, parents typically agree to try the diet. If any celiac IgA tests are positive (see "Testing for Celiac Disease," page 167), a more detailed analysis for celiac disease is done (but this is rare).

The challenge arises when the tests are normal. In such cases, we consider other causes of the chronic symptoms and perhaps perform more tests to evaluate these other causes. But we also encourage these families to commit to going gluten-free to rule out the diagnosis because blood tests *can* be falsely normal. Sometimes the diet trial provides the answer, and sometimes it does not. But it's a crucial step. To allow an infant or child to continue to suffer with chronic and severe symptoms isn't right, and the damage gluten does to the immune, intestinal, and nervous systems at a time of life when these systems are developing and maturing can have lifelong consequences. Undiagnosed and untreated gluten sensitivity can cause irreversible harm if it goes unchecked. Admittedly, gluten sensitivity isn't common, but it is growing. A gluten-free trial, if recommended by your doctor, is the gold standard in diagnosing non-celiac gluten sensitivity.

GLUTEN SENSITIVITY IS INHERITED

We know that celiac disease runs in families; research demonstrates that about 5 percent of children will have it if a parent does. What about non-celiac gluten sensitivity? During our

(continued)

conversations with parents regarding their child's gluten sensitivity, we are continually amazed at how often we hear a mom say, "Hmmm. That's interesting, because *I'm* sensitive to gluten as well." Or, "His father is on a gluten-free diet and he feels much better." Gluten sensitivity does run in families, but the exact percentage is unknown. If a parent is known to be sensitive, many doctors will advise that the children remain gluten-free during the first few years of life, when the immune and neurological systems are developing. This gives you the opportunity to prevent the behavioral, developmental, and allergic problems before they even begin. Gluten can be introduced later in a child's life, as he or she begins exploring foods outside the home. Appropriate testing can be done at a later age as well.

There may be a problem with this advice, however. Some research has shown that exposure to allergenic foods early in life might actually *prevent* later development of allergies. One recent study demonstrated that moms who routinely ate gluten, peanuts, and milk products during pregnancy had children with fewer allergies. This suggests that early exposure can help a person become more tolerant of allergenic foods. For families *without* a history of gluten sensitivity, it may be important to allow some gluten routinely during young childhood, if it's tolerated.

For families *with* sensitivity, this research is conflicting. One study showed that delaying gluten introduction until twelve months of age in infants with a genetic risk of celiac disease (severe gluten allergy) reduced the chance of subsequent celiac disease compared with starting gluten at six months of age. However, another study in families with celiac disease showed that introducing small quantities of gluten between four and seven months of age, particularly in breastfed infants, reduced that baby's risk of eventually developing the disease, and waiting *past* seven months to introduce gluten increased the risk.

There are three points on which researchers do agree: (1) allowing large amounts of gluten during infancy seems to increase risk,

(2) introducing gluten while still breastfeeding seems to be protective, and (3) we don't yet know what the best time is to introduce gluten.

The best compromise for gluten-sensitive families may be to keep an infant mostly gluten-free but allow occasional exposure around six months of age to provide some benefit in preventing later sensitivity. Obtain some products made with ancient strains of wheat, like einkorn and emmer (see page 153); feed some standard wheat foods as well on occasion. If allergic symptoms are seen, stricter adherence to the gluten-free diet may be needed for that infant. Discuss your unique situation and family history with your doctor.

CELIAC DISEASE: GLUTEN SENSITIVITY AT ITS WORST

Celiac disease (CD) is an extreme autoimmune reaction to gluten. Fortunately, CD only affects 1 percent of the population. While most of you who are reading this won't have to worry about celiac disease, it is on the rise. One study has demonstrated a fourfold increase over the last fifty years. A 2010 Canadian study revealed a tenfold rise in the disease in children between 1998 and 2007. For those who do suffer from CD, the negative impact gluten has on almost every part of the body can be severe. Receiving an accurate and timely diagnosis is crucial, so that diet and healing can begin. Here is what you need to know about diagnosing and treating celiac disease.

Unique Immune Response to Gluten

For those with CD, the immune reaction to gluten is far worse than the general allergic reaction you've read about with other foods. A person with CD is born with a specific genetically programmed sensitivity to gluten. Once gluten is digested into gliadin and other protein fragments, the T lymphocytes attack these proteins and create IgA and IgG antibodies against them (normal allergic reactions, as you remember, generate IgE antibodies). If only it ended there. Unfortunately, the T lymphocytes also create IgA and IgG antibodies that attack three specific body tissues: tissue transglutaminase, an enzyme in the intestinal lining that helps digest gluten; endomysium, a protein within the muscular layers of the intestines; and reticulin, fibers that provide strength and structure to numerous body organs. We know that the IgA antibodies are a definite indication of severe celiac sensitivity; IgG reactions are less significant but do indicate sensitivity. In addition to the antibodies, some T lymphocytes release cytokines and enzymes that directly damage the cells of the intestinal lining. This is why CD is considered an autoimmune disorder, not an allergic one. Your body's immune system turns against your own body.

Symptoms of Celiac Disease

CD has two types of presentations. One is obvious, but the other is subtle:

Classic symptoms. Approximately 50 percent of sufferers will present with the classic signs of the disease: abdominal pain, cramping, bloating, diarrhea, and weight loss. If the disease goes unchecked for too long, lab work will reveal deficiencies in folate, iron, zinc, protein, fat, and vitamins A, D, E, and K.

Modern symptoms. Due to changes in the genetic structure of modern wheat, the immune system now reacts differently to gluten in the other 50 percent of patients. GI symptoms may not be apparent at all or may come decades into the disease. Instead, these patients have a variety of the following symptoms:

- Neurological complaints, such as migraine headaches, dizziness and loss of coordination, or numbness in the arms or legs
- Arthritis and other types of chronic pain
- Psychiatric signs like dementia, impaired focus, depression, and even psychosis
- Rashes (see page 156), particularly dermatitis herpetiformis
- Chronic fatigue syndrome
- Anemia
- Infertility
- Short stature in kids
- Abdominal pain without diarrhea
- Obesity (due to the carbohydrate overload of wheat)

Testing for Celiac Disease

In our practice, we now routinely test all patients with chronic GI symptoms. We also test children with developmental delays, behavioral disorders, and neurological problems. We rarely find actual CD, but we do discover gluten sensitivity in some patients. Here are the available tests (all are blood tests, unless indicated otherwise), which measure the autoimmune reactions to gluten described above:

Tissue transglutaminase IgA antibody (tTG). This new test measures the immune system's IgA reaction to this intestinal enzyme. This is now considered the most accurate blood indicator of CD and will be positive in virtually all cases. IgG can also be tested, but it isn't considered as significant in CD. A drawback of this test, however, is that it is often negative in early CD, before enough intestinal damage has occurred to create a high tTG antibody response.

Endomysial IgA antibody. This is an older test that measures the immune system's IgA reaction to this intestinal muscle protein.

This was previously considered the gold standard blood test, but most experts now believe that tTG is a better test, and many no longer test for both antibodies.

Gliadin (deamidated) IgA antibody. This test measures the IgA reaction to the gliadin protein (one of the proteins that make up gluten). An older version of the test measured IgA antibodies to *all* the gliadin proteins. The newer version detects only IgA antibodies to the *deamidated* gliadin protein. The reason for this change is that when gluten is digested in CD, the resulting gliadin protein undergoes a further step called deamidation, meaning an amide molecule is removed. It is thought that only the deamidated form of gliadin is responsible for CD; the immune response to the other gliadin proteins may suggest sensitivity to gluten, but not to a degree that would indicate CD. Researchers thought that the older version, which was revealing CD in a higher percentage of people, was revealing a high number of false positive results (showing an abnormal result in people who do not actually have CD). Doctors worried that people were being overdiagnosed with CD. This new test, therefore, is intended to reveal only those people who are truly highly sensitive to gluten (or to the deamidated portion of the gliadin protein) to a degree that could lead to CD. The gliadin *IgG* antibody test for non-celiac gluten sensitivity, discussed on page 161, has also been changed to measure only the deamidated portions of the reaction. The obvious downside of these new deaminated tests is that they miss many people who have non-celiac gluten sensitivity. Many sufferers are being tested with the new test and are being told they are not gluten-sensitive when, in fact, they may be. Few labs offer the old version of the gliadin test (called a native gliadin antibody test, for both IgG and IgA reactions to gliadin); if your doctor can arrange it, it is a more practical marker for gluten sensitivity, but must be arranged through a specialty lab. Finally, neither version of the test is 100 percent accurate: even some people with CD won't register a positive native or deamidated gliadin test.

Reticulin IgA antibody. This older test measures IgA response to this fibrous tissue (IgG can also be tested). Because it is positive in only some people with CD, it isn't usually tested anymore.

Total IgA antibody. This should be measured along with any gluten-specific IgA antibody test. This is because some people have very low IgA antibodies in general; such people won't generate IgA antibodies against gluten, even if they have CD. Gluten IgA testing is therefore inaccurate in such people. A normal total IgA result confirms that the patient is capable of reacting to gluten, thus confirming that the tests are accurate.

Note: All of the above tests will be accurate only for people who are eating gluten. Those who have been on a gluten-free diet for a few months or more will likely show normal test results.

Genetic testing (HLA-DQ). Two genes show up in over 90 percent of people with CD: HLA-DQ2 and -DQ8. They are partly responsible for programming the autoimmune reaction in the T lymphocytes. Testing for the presence of these genes helps determine a person's genetic risk of developing CD. But there's a drawback to the test: almost half of our population has at least one of these two genes. So the test may be useful in predicting the risk of CD in those with both gene markers, and it may encourage such people to go gluten-free. But it certainly is *not* a tool that is used to make a diagnosis of CD.

Intestinal biopsy. Performed by a GI specialist, this procedure directly detects gluten-induced damage to the intestinal lining and is considered the most accurate way to diagnose CD. A patient must be eating gluten for the test to be valid. Because CD is a lifelong condition with severe consequences if left untreated, GI specialists strongly recommend this confirmatory procedure before committing to a life without gluten.

Diagnosing Celiac Disease

The diagnosis of celiac disease is based solely on test results. One of the primary tests, either IgA antibody or intestinal biopsy, has to be positive for a person to receive the diagnosis. The only exception to this rule is someone who very clearly suffers from severe gluten-associated symptoms with exposure and has obvious relief from elimination, but has normal test results. But this scenario is rare.

The steps taken to make the diagnosis of CD are the same as with any other food sensitivity disorder: symptoms suggest a problem and tests are done to evaluate the cause. A CD diagnosis is usually "stumbled upon" when a doctor is running tests to evaluate multiple food allergies and sensitivities in a patient with chronic intestinal, immune, allergic, or neurological symptoms. Rarely does a doctor decide to look only for CD in such patients. The first clue to diagnosis is usually a positive CD blood test during such extensive work-ups.

Controversy exists as to whether or not people with a positive blood test for celiac disease should undergo intestinal biopsy before beginning a gluten-free life. Most GI specialists say yes, confirm the diagnosis before making such a drastic change. We disagree. Here's why: If you have symptoms, and a blood test reveals that CD is likely, you really have no choice but to try to go gluten-free. If you wait and do an intestinal biopsy first, the result won't change what you should do. If the biopsy is *abnormal,* you go gluten-free. If the biopsy is *normal,* you should still go gluten-free because the blood test revealed a likely problem and the biopsy may have missed it. This is particularly true in children, as a biopsy is invasive and sedation carries risks. The procedure is much better tolerated by adults. In our practice, any abnormal IgA gluten test buys that patient a gluten-free diet.

The decision to do a biopsy can easily be made later if a person's symptoms don't improve on a gluten-free diet. At that point, gluten is reintroduced and a biopsy is done, not only to check for celiac disease, but to test for a variety of other chronic intestinal conditions as well. But the hope is that you'll feel better on the diet and no biopsy will be needed.

STARTING A GLUTEN-FREE DIET

You've hemmed and hawed. You've procrastinated. You've lived in denial that gluten may be a problem. But now you're ready to make the leap. We think you'll be surprised at how easy it is to go gluten-free. Or how easy it is to get *started* on the diet. Making a *long-term* commitment to living gluten-free, even when you realize the diet actually helps, is admittedly a greater challenge. My family started a gluten-free diet about nine months before we began this book. By the time of publication it will have been over two years. It has been easy to control gluten at home. Going out to eat is what we found most challenging at first. But we've since figured it out, and we are enjoying the health benefits today. Here is our guide to getting started.

Step One: Understand the Basics of What to Avoid

Gluten is a protein in wheat (all forms, including bulgur, durum, graham, Kamut, semolina, and spelt), rye, barley, and triticale. You therefore have to avoid all bread, cereal, pasta, baked goods, and prepared foods that contain these grains. But it isn't always this obvious; here is a list of the many sources of gluten that a rookie might not recognize:

Common Sources of Gluten

Biscuits	Graham crackers	Pizza
Blue cheese crumbles	Gravy	Salad dressing
Bran	Hot dogs	Sausage
Candy and candy bars	Imitation meats	Commercial Seasonings
	Jerky	
Condiments	Macaroni	Soups
Couscous	Matzo	Sprouted wheat/barley
Crackers	Meatballs	Tabbouleh (tabouli)
Croutons	Noodles	Teriyaki and other sauces
Dumplings	Oats (from cross-contamination)	
Farina		Wheat germ

These items all contain gluten unless specifically made and labeled gluten-free.

ALCOHOL AND GLUTEN

Some distilled alcohol is made from gluten grains. These include whiskey, vodka, and gin (unless made from a nongluten source, like potato vodka). However, most experts agree that the distillation process removes all gluten proteins, so the final product should be gluten-free (although it won't be labeled as such). Beer, on the other hand, does contain gluten, unless made and labeled gluten-free. Distilled alcohols that are not made from gluten grains include virtually all rums and tequilas (unless flavored with a gluten ingredient), as well as wine; these can be enjoyed responsibly by adults.

Step Two: Understand What You Can Eat

Now for the good news. There are many tasty options that will make your diet complete. Flour made from the following sources can allow you to enjoy your pasta, crackers, pizza, bread, and other baked goods:

Almonds (and other nuts)	Corn	Quinoa
	Flax	Rice
Amaranth	Millet	Rhubarb
Arrowroot	Oats (if labeled gluten-free)*	Sorghum
Beans (like garbanzo)		Soy
Buckwheat	Peas	Tapioca
Chia	Potatoes	Teff

* Note: Oats are gluten-free in nature but often become contaminated during harvesting and processing. Oats are safe and healthy if labeled gluten-free.

Step Three: Don't Buy Gluten-Free Foods Yet

When you first go gluten-free, don't start buying a cupboardful of gluten-free products. Sounds like unusual advice for this section, but hear us out. Gluten-free replacement foods taste very different from their counterparts. Take bread, for example. Most gluten-free bread tastes, well, not like the bread you are accustomed to: it's firm, dry, and generally flavorless. Spare yourself the disappointment. You'll hopefully find a decent-tasting bread later on (we finally did!). For now, simply stop eating bread. Ditto for many snack foods, like crackers, pretzels, and some cookies. This is especially true for children: when they're presented with gluten-free snack foods after years of yummy, bready, melt-in-your-mouth snacks, you'll have a rebellion on your hands. Kids will reject these changes. You're trying to get your family motivated to follow the new lifestyle, and you don't need bad-tasting food weighing you down.

Instead, during the first month or two of the new diet, simply stop eating foods with gluten without trying to replace them. Run out of each snack food. Your child may ask you when you're going to buy more of her favorite crackers, but soon the out-of-sight, out-of-mind principle will set in. Your young kids don't even have to know you are going gluten-free. After a few months, you will have fun trying healthier replacements for all the foods you miss the most, and your kids will be more likely to accept them once the old gluten tastes have been out of their mouths for a while. You'll buy some foods that taste like cardboard, but you'll find many that are surprisingly tasty. Read online reviews and get advice from veteran friends about which brands get it right. On my new website, DrBobsDaily.com, I post some of my family's favorite finds, including some delicious breads, cereals, and even a replacement for Oreo cookies that you won't believe.

CHERYL SEARS'S SECRET GLUTEN-FREE FLOUR MIX

In her quest to find the perfect flour replacement for her family-famous pancakes and waffles and her neighborhood-famous chocolate chip cookies, Dr. Bob's wife searched high and low for a replacement flour that didn't taste gluten-free. She couldn't find one. Some made the batter too runny, and some were too goopy. So she mixed and matched several brands until she developed a flour that baked well and tasted great. In fact, her chocolate cake and pumpkin bread are even moister than before. For every cup of flour in a recipe, she substitutes the following (which are blends of rice, potato, tapioca, sorghum, almond, and arrowroot):

- Pamela's Artisan Flour Blend — 1/2 cup plus 1/8 cup
- Trader Joe's Baker Josef's Gluten Free All Purpose Flour — 1/4 cup
- Any almond flour — 1/8 cup
- As an added trick to improve flavor, she adds an extra teaspoon of vanilla to any baked recipe, even if vanilla isn't in the ingredients list.

> • To thicken the final product a bit, as she needs to do for her chocolate chip cookies, she adds a tiny bit more Pamela's and a bit less almond. I know that "bits" aren't an actual measurement, but Cheryl is still artfully playing with the mix (as it should be with baking) and doesn't have it down to a science yet. Does any good baker?

Step Four: Make Changes Gradually

Don't instantly go hard-core gluten-free. The chemical withdrawal from gluten may cause mood swings and increase your craving. Instead, allow yourself and your family about a month to reach your goal. Let your child have those last few team treats after the soccer game, or birthday cake at the party. Enjoy a last night out at your favorite Italian restaurant. Don't scan every label and live in fear of gluten contamination at first; save that for later. Here are some ways to phase out of wheat and gluten, without worrying about how to replace them just yet:

Dinner. First off, stop serving bread with dinner and don't make any pasta for a few weeks. Instead, dinner should be meat, poultry, fish, and vegetables.

Breakfast and lunch. Next you tackle the other meals. No more wheat-based cereal, toast, bagels, or English muffins for breakfast. Eggs, breakfast meats, rice-based and other nongluten cereals, and oatmeal should become the norm. Homemade waffles and pancakes can eventually follow, as you begin to experiment with gluten-free flour mixes. Lunch will have no more bread or snack crackers. Hot-lunch menus at school will offer some gluten-free choices that are decent (and some that are *not*).

Snacks. Snack time can revolve around nuts, trail mix, fruit, veggies dipped in hummus, and apples dipped in peanut butter. Finish off some of the favorite gluten snacks in the cupboard.

Dessert. Enjoy the last servings of your favorite baked treats, then visit your local gluten-free bakery and learn what it has to offer. Start baking your own specialties with gluten-free flour blends (see box on page 174) and enjoy! Luckily, ice cream is gluten-free.

Remember, this first month isn't about finding equivalent-tasting replacement foods. It's more about simply going wheat-free at first and allowing your body to adjust to the changes.

Step Five: Don't Overload on Gluten-Free Carbs

A common mistake many people make is to replace gluten with meals full of rice, corn, potato, and other gluten-free grains and starches. The result is that many people end up eating even *more* carbs than when they were on a regular diet. The metabolic effects of this carb overload may be as unhealthy as wheat overload. Also, these extra starchy carbs are a banquet for intestinal bacteria. As you read in Chapter 1, the healthy probiotic germs that thrive in our intestines are in a constant battle with unhealthy bacteria and yeast. Carb overload feeds the unhealthy germs, which leads to unhealthy immune imbalance in the gut and the rest of the body. This is, in part, why we advise against buying many gluten-free replacement foods early in the diet. In Chapter 14, we present some healthier, low-carb approaches to going GF. In time, you will be able to enjoy carbs again, after the gut has had time to heal.

Step Six: Go 100 Percent Gluten-Free

To realize the complete benefits of going gluten-free, you'll need to commit to it for at least a few months. Experts believe that it can take that long for all traces of gluten and its effects to leave the body. Many will see benefits right away; if you don't, hang in there for as long as you can. There are anecdotal reports of some people seeing major benefits after six months or more.

You'll need to achieve a 100 percent gluten-free lifestyle to best evaluate whether or not the diet is helping you. If you see benefits from being *mostly* gluten-free, you should see what happens with absolutely *no* gluten. If you don't see benefits from reducing gluten, this may be because you are extremely sensitive and you won't see changes until you are completely free.

You don't have to remain 100 percent gluten-free forever. If you see no benefit at all, you can reintroduce gluten and explore other causes of your chronic symptoms. If you *do* see benefits, remain as gluten-free as you can for a while, then begin experimenting to see if you can tolerate a certain amount of gluten. See the section on page 185 for more information.

This book provides an introduction to going gluten-free. If you decide that the diet is a success, you should seek out additional resources for ways to optimize your new lifestyle. There are many books and online sources of information that will teach you everything you need to know. Here are a few key tips:

Label reading. It's getting easier and easier to find gluten on food labels. All foods that are marketed as gluten-free will say so very clearly on the front of the label. But some manufacturers don't want to make it obvious for fear of scaring away gluten eaters, to whom *gluten-free* is synonymous with *taste-free*. Look at the end of the ingredients list; most labels will list the allergens that are contained in the product, such as nuts, milk, eggs, and wheat. If wheat is listed there, you don't have to bother reading all of the ingredients. If you don't see wheat, then it's *probably* gluten-free; scan the entire ingredient list just to be sure. You may see the phrase *may contain wheat, manufactured on equipment also used to process wheat,* or other such phrases. These foods don't intentionally have wheat or gluten and are usually fine for those of us who are not severely sensitive. We now eat the "may contain" foods, as long as gluten isn't actually listed as an ingredient. But low levels of gluten can inadvertently contaminate such foods, and these may not be safe for those with celiac disease. You should carefully watch for reactions to such foods and determine your own level of sensitivity.

Here are some nonobvious sources of gluten on labels:

- Brewer's yeast
- Food starch
- Inulin
- Malt (syrup, extract, vinegar, flavoring)
- Smoked flavoring
- Soy sauce (usually made with wheat)
- Vegetable protein
- Vegetable starch

Eating out without fear. My family's first few times eating out were a little scary; we were so worried about gluten contamination that we didn't even enjoy our meals. We learned pretty quickly never to attempt a gluten-free meal at a restaurant that wasn't set up for it. Now we look online or call ahead and ask if the establishment has a separate gluten-free menu. This means that instead of just removing gluten ingredients (and the flavor) from dishes that really should have gluten, a restaurant has some well-thought-out, delicious meals for us to choose from. Don't try to put together your own gluten-free meal off a regular menu; you'll likely be disappointed in the lack of choices and flavor.

Looking for a fast meal? Some fast-food restaurants have a dedicated fryer for their fries (they don't fry any breaded items in the same fryer), so you can enjoy them as an occasional treat. Lettuce-wrapped burgers or chicken are a little messy, but they can still hit the spot. Learn which establishments in your town offer this option. Of course, you shouldn't really be eating at such places too often anyway.

Here are a few hidden sources of gluten that you may encounter in a restaurant if you aren't careful:

- Meatballs and some sausages (they may contain bread or flour)
- Blue cheese crumbles on salad (often cultured on wheat or mixed with flour)
- Fries or tortilla chips fried in oil that is used to fry breaded foods
- Salad dressing
- Chicken dishes (they often use flour)
- Soy or teriyaki sauce
- Some condiments, like BBQ sauce and mustard

Try not to be a gluten snob—someone who expects every restaurant to cater to gluten-free customers and gets all huffy when the waiter doesn't even know what gluten is. The day will come when you can enjoy gluten-free meals pretty much everywhere. Meanwhile, it's your own responsibility to know what you are doing, and to find restaurants that provide a good meal. My wife and I found ourselves at a fund-raising banquet that was serving breaded chicken breast. So we asked for a gluten-free version, and we got chicken breast with…well, just chicken breast—no seasoning or flavor at all. And there was no gluten-free dressing for our salad. Although slightly disappointed, we just smiled at each other, knowing that we chose this diet for our health, and that the world doesn't need to bow and scrape to our health needs.

Shopping. Plan to spend about three times as long at the grocery store on your first few gluten-free shopping trips. You may want to leave young children at home, because you'll need to focus. We suggest you start with your local health food grocery store; these stores will have a large gluten-free section, and they will likely have easy-to-spot gluten-free labels on other items scattered around the store. Be prepared for some disappointment as you discover some foods that taste like cardboard. But food makers have begun to excel at gluten-free cooking, and you'll find plenty of your favorite foods in a gluten-free form that you and your family can enjoy. Small groceries that are completely dedicated to gluten-free shopping are now opening up around the country; you will be amazed at all the choices these offer you. Online retailers are another useful resource, and you can read reviews to guide your selections.

GOING ON VACATION? CALL AND PLAN AHEAD

It just so happened that our ten-day Walt Disney World family vacation came a few months into our gluten-free lifestyle. We were a little stressed about making things work, thinking there was no way we could eat out at six different amusement parks without contamination. Boy, were we surprised! Disney had gone the extra mile by providing delicious gluten-free choices at several restaurants in every park. These options are even labeled on the park maps, and Disney employees are well versed in gluten-free eating. We had a fantastic seasoned steak at one restaurant, and the kids still talk about it today. Investigate your vacation destination before you embark. You may find it easier than you think.

MISCONCEPTIONS ABOUT THE GLUTEN-FREE DIET

The gluten-free craze has given rise to many myths and misconceptions. Some proponents rave that everyone should go gluten-free. Many in the medical establishment warn against it unless a definitive diagnosis has been made. Food companies are scrambling to rise to the top of the gluten-free food chain with delicious offerings. Books, magazines, organizations, and websites are popping up left and right with advice for the growing body of disciples. This influx of ideas and information has led to some misconceptions that we would like to address here:

Gluten-free must be all or nothing. Many who espouse the gluten-free diet preach that you must be absolutely 100 percent gluten-free always, or your body will suffer severe consequences. They say that even a tiny exposure will unleash the fury of the immune system for months to come. We agree that this is certainly true for those with celiac disease; the autoimmune response to gluten, even in small quantities, can have immediately noticeable effects as well as underlying immune and neurological consequences. But CD sufferers are the only group in which we know this to be true. For those with non-celiac gluten sensitivity, or wheat allergy, the consequences are probably far less dire and will vary from person to person. Little research exists on tolerance levels for this group; we don't know how careful you must be and what the long-term consequences are of low-level exposure because true, systematic research is still lacking. Does exposure cause a metabolic and immune reaction that could go unnoticed, only to create severe consequences years later? Or will you simply experience some temporary and minor symptoms that will pass without any lasting internal effects? Do you enjoy that occasional slice of pizza and accept the fact that you'll feel crummy for a day or two (it may be worth it), or will such infractions slowly eat away at your insides without your knowing it?

The problem is that many people take what we know about CD and apply it to everyone with gluten sensitivity. Such people would therefore advise remaining 100 percent gluten-free all the time. But most information and advice in this area is mainly theoretical at this time. Therefore, the answers to these questions must be approached on a case-by-case basis. You will see for yourself whether you or your children feel any benefits during your initial months on the diet, and whether or not you have any noticeable symptoms when you eat some gluten (see section on "Reintroducing Wheat and Gluten" below). If you do, you should be as gluten-free as you can be, for as long as you can be. Research will provide us with more guidance in the years to come.

My family had an eye-opening experience when my wife and child ate some licorice during our annual gingerbread house–making contest, not suspecting that licorice would contain wheat. I saw my child taking his second bite and rushed in to stop him. He then panicked, started crying, and moaned that he'd messed up and now his body had to start all over on the diet. It seems we had educated him a little too thoroughly on how important it was for him to be gluten-free. We had to reassure him that one little bite wouldn't cause any harm. He seemed totally fine that night and the following day, and the incident was soon forgotten.

Did that one bite cause our son some sort of internal harm that we can't measure? We'll never know. We don't even know if he really has gluten sensitivity in the first place. He had a positive IgG result for gluten (see page 160), but that isn't a definitive test. We are mainly doing the diet for autoimmune health (he has autoimmune thyroid disease). The chronic pimply rash on his arms has gone away, and he's thinned out a little. But that's all we have been able to notice. If he is sensitive, his sensitivity is probably mild. A few years from now we will likely allow some gluten back into his life and see how his thyroid health manages it. But I share this story so that you'll be aware that accidents can happen, and that you don't have to freak out over them unless you know that gluten causes you harm.

We see a subset of patients who react severely to gluten, and those are our patients with autism. For some of these kids, a gluten meal causes days to weeks of worsened behavior. Let's say Grandma is watching little Joey and decides to give him a cupcake because his parents are so "mean" with their "gluten-free fad." Wham! Most of Joey's autism symptoms flare up for weeks. Thanks, Grandma. Parents know their children the best. It's important that other family members, friends, and teachers listen to, and respect, your diet choices.

The gluten-free diet is deficient in essential nutrients. This misconception is ignorance at its best—or worst. Wheat does not contain a single nutrient that can't be easily found in most other foods. Yet you will hear some medical professionals warn that the diet can cause deficiencies in various vitamins, iron, and protein. I have seen many children with chronic GI problems who needed to go gluten-free, but who were warned by other doctors not to do so because of such fears. Granted, a child who is hooked on wheat carbs could be a little undernourished as he rejects your attempts to feed him more meats, fish, eggs, nuts, fruits, and veggies. But only temporarily. As your child's diet expands again and gluten-free favorites are discovered, nutrition will return to normal, and it will likely be even better. Also, the healing for the GI and immune systems will add even more benefits to your child's health.

The only scenario in which we have seen a child become malnourished on a gluten-free diet is in a few cases of autism. Some of these kids have severe oral aversions to any change in diet, and they may go many days without eating until you give in and let them eat their favorites again. But this is a very small minority. We have seen most kids with autism show amazing improvements on the diet, if and when they are able to accept it.

Gluten-free foods cost too much. If you're buying gluten-free foods, expect to pay more for most of them. As they become more popular, prices may come down. But it's only costly if you try to find replacements for all your carb-laden foods: pasta, cereal, bread, crackers, snacks, and cookies. As you will learn later in this book, eating low-carb is a healthier choice for those with chronic allergies and inflammation. So you may not find yourself buying many of these gluten-free replacement foods.

Gluten-free diets are dangerous because of arsenic. This is partly true, in that arsenic in the soil has a particular affinity for rice, and rice crops absorb more arsenic than other grains do. Therefore, anyone who eats a high-rice diet (whether gluten-free or not) will ingest more arsenic. Because some gluten-free foods are made with rice, this diet may increase exposure. That's the true part of the statement. But the diet does not expose anyone to dangerous levels of arsenic. This concern was first discovered about ten years ago, and the initial worry was that infants who were given organic formulas containing brown-rice syrup would ingest too much arsenic. Since that time, the FDA and other research organizations have continued to study this problem; you can read updates on FDA.gov. The amount of arsenic in rice is extremely low, and we can safely enjoy it in moderate amounts. Vary the diet with several nongluten grains, in addition to rice, to limit arsenic. But this worry is not an accurate reason to avoid being gluten-free if you need, or want, to be. We suspect that this concern is being promoted by food growers and manufacturers who are trying to steer people away from gluten-free choices and back to their own wheat-based products.

WHAT TO DO IF YOU'VE BEEN "GLUTENED"

Some anecdotal reports show that two remedies *may* help accidental ingestion: activated charcoal (available over-the-counter at any drugstore) and digestive enzymes (available online and at health food and vitamin stores). If you learn that gluten does negatively affect you, keep these remedies on hand and take as directed as soon as you can.

REINTRODUCING WHEAT AND GLUTEN

Anyone who has been gluten-free for a while will eventually become curious about how gluten-free they really have to be.

If your wheat or gluten symptoms were severe, and you see great results from being gluten-free, don't be in a hurry to reintroduce. Remain free for as long as you can, even for several years, if the initial changes were dramatic. If that was not the case for you—either the severity or the improvement—reintroduce sooner.

I plan to remain mostly gluten-free for the rest of my life, but I do plan to test my limits in a few years to see whether I can tolerate some wheat without losing my breath. Many of you will wish to do the same, and we believe that you eventually should, unless you've been diagnosed with celiac disease.

Go Slow

We recommend you try half a serving of a food you miss the most for breakfast. This gives you all day to observe how you or your child feels. To allow it to sink in, don't eat any more gluten for at least a week. If you don't notice any problems, continue this weekly treat (and go for a full serving) for a month. If all is well, enjoy twice-weekly meals that include gluten. Continue to expand the diet as long as you don't notice any problems. Be sure to observe for GI symptoms, rash, fatigue, or any other chronic symptom that you initially attributed to gluten. If you truly are very sensitive, you may experience food poisoning symptoms: vomiting, abdominal pain, and diarrhea. If any *new* symptom develops that you didn't experience with gluten before, that may be significant too.

Instead of jumping right into regular wheat, consider buying foods made with ancient wheat grains, such as einkorn or emmer, which are much lower in gluten and have not undergone genetic expansion over the centuries.

If at any time in this process you notice problems, resume gluten-free living again, this time for a longer period (perhaps years). You can decide down the road when to go off the diet.

Repeat Allergy Tests

If you had abnormal wheat or gluten test results before the diet, we recommend you repeat the tests before you start gluten again. It is useful to see whether the tests turn normal when you're off gluten, and most of them should. If you successfully reintroduce gluten and believe you see no problems from it, you can then get blood work done to make sure your gluten tests remain normal. There is no standard period you must wait, so you should discuss this with your health care provider. If your tests were initially normal, there is little value in repeating the tests again, unless recommended by a doctor.

One exception to this rule is as follows: if the only gluten or wheat test that was initially abnormal was an IgG level specific to wheat or gluten (see page 160), retesting this may not be useful. IgG levels may stay elevated for years, even on the diet. Research has not yet determined how useful IgG levels are as a tool to monitor people on and off the diet.

Beware of Cravings

If you find that eating wheat and gluten again causes unusual cravings for more and more, this may be a sign that you are feeling the effects of gluteomorphin (see page 158). Even if you don't experience any negative symptoms that indicate you still need the diet, this druglike effect may be indication enough that gluten isn't right for you.

KEEP UP TO DATE

More accurate information on wheat and gluten sensitivity will continue to emerge in the coming years. Periodically update yourself by reading online and asking a knowledgeable doctor for any new information. On DrBobsDaily.com I will provide updates and make gluten-free product recommendations as my family and I discover more delicious foods.

9

Other Food Allergies: Peanuts, Tree Nuts, Fish, Shellfish, Eggs, Soy, Corn, and Chemical Additives

Chapter 6 introduced you to food allergies and sensitivities in general. You've since examined milk and wheat as the most common culprits. But there are other foods that deserve their moment in the spotlight as well: peanuts, tree nuts, fish (and shellfish), eggs, and soy. These eight foods are responsible for about 90 percent of food allergies. This chapter presents some additional details on each and provides guidance on diagnosis and treatment. Corn allergy and behavioral sensitivity are also a growing problem. And some chemicals that are added to foods can trigger an allergic or sensitive reaction, including MSG, food coloring, and other artificial ingredients. These issues are explored in this chapter as well.

We should note that all allergic disorders are on the rise in developed countries, so the increasing incidence of food allergy is likely due to many environmental and nutritional factors in modernized countries (detailed on page 12). Food allergies are rare in many developing countries, where children grow up in far less sterile environments than in developed countries. This lends credibility to the hygiene hypothesis, which holds that exposure to the outdoors, animals, dirt, and germs (things our infants in the United States experience far less of) may actually improve the immune system and reduce allergies.

PEANUT ALLERGY

After milk and wheat, peanuts probably cause the next most common food allergy. But peanuts' potential to cause a severe anaphylactic reaction is far greater than that of wheat or milk. And this is a growing problem. Research has shown that peanut allergy almost tripled between 1997 and 2008. The reason for this rise is unclear, but it may be due in part to the genetic modification of soybeans in our American culture. Peanuts belong to the same family of foods as soybeans (peanuts are not related to tree nuts; instead, they are a member of the legume family, which includes soybeans, lentils, peas, and other beans). More than 90 percent of the soy used in the United States is genetically modified, a process that first began in 1996. During these last two decades, soy has become an additive in an ever-increasing list of food and other products. The latest generation of children has essentially grown up with almost daily exposure to modified soy. The theory is that children are becoming sensitive to this artificial soy, and that, in turn, is making them cross-react to peanuts. Is it coincidence that peanut allergy and soy allergy have both risen dramatically since 1996? It isn't clear. This theory is explored in more detail in a very interesting book, *The Unhealthy Truth* by Robyn O'Brien. She uncovers some alarming information about the food industry and GMO foods that is worth reading.

If you or someone in your family has been diagnosed with peanut allergy, or you suspect an allergy, Chapter 6 covered what you need to know about allergy testing, and Chapter 11, "Anaphylaxis: From Mild Hives to Life-Threatening Allergic Reactions," demonstrates how you should be prepared to treat an allergic reaction. Those with diagnosed peanut allergy should definitely carry an epinephrine injection for self-administration in case of an emergency. In this section, we expand on what you need to know to best avoid exposure to peanuts.

How to Avoid Peanut Exposure

Because of the high potential for anaphylaxis (severe, life-threatening allergic reaction), those with peanut allergy must be particularly careful. Here are some obvious and not-so-obvious sources to watch out for:

Cross-contamination. Read labels carefully, and avoid any foods that are labeled with the phrase *may contain peanuts* or *made in a facility which uses peanuts*. The dust from ground peanuts can easily travel through the air and contaminate nearby foods or remain on shared equipment.

Peanut oil. Because it is the protein component of peanuts that triggers the allergy, experts now believe that *highly refined* peanut oil is safe for most allergic people to eat, as it shouldn't contain any protein. Cold-pressed, expelled, or extruded oil is not as pure and should not be consumed by most people with peanut allergy. Consult with your allergy specialist for an opinion specific to your situation.

Hiding places. Peanuts can show up in unexpected places, such as sauces, desserts, and various dishes in certain cuisines (particularly Asian, Mexican, and African). Here are foods or environments to be aware of that aren't so obvious:

- Candy
- Chocolate bars
- Cookies
- Chopped peanuts at ice cream or frozen yogurt parlors
- Cereals
- Sauces
- Marinades
- Various Asian dishes
- Peanut sauce
- Salad bars with chopped peanuts
- Trail mix
- Granola bars and energy bars
- Chili, soups, or gravies, especially at restaurants
- Other nut butters that may be made on shared equipment
- *Mole* sauce (used in Mexican dishes)

Desensitization Therapy

Unlike many other allergies, peanut allergy does not yet have a protocol for using allergy shots to eliminate the allergy (nor do many other food allergies). However, some newly developed oral challenge protocols specifically for peanuts look promising. Starting with very small quantities, gradually escalating doses of peanuts are eaten in an allergist's office every day, and the patient is monitored for reactions, with emergency medication on standby. If tolerated, the process may be continued at home, with periodic dose increases at the doctor's office. Sublingual immunotherapy, using allergen tablets that dissolve under the tongue, is also being investigated for peanuts and may become available in the coming years.

Component Allergy Testing

Introduced on page 118, this new blood test from the Immuno-CAP company measures allergy to five different peanut proteins, labeled as Ara h 1, 2, 3, 8, and 9. Allergy to Ara h 1 through 3 causes the worst allergic reactions. Severity of reaction to Ara h 9 varies, and allergy to only Ara h 8 tends to cause the mildest reaction and is unlikely to trigger anaphylaxis. Knowing such results can help you plan how careful you need to be around peanuts and whether or not to carry an epinephrine injector.

Common Questions

Do people outgrow peanut allergy? Children who are diagnosed with peanut allergy have a 20 to 25 percent chance of outgrowing the allergy by the time they reach the teen years. Oral desensitization therapy may increase this chance. On the other hand, adults who develop the allergy *as adults* are unlikely to outgrow it.

How can I prevent peanut allergy in my children? Opinions on this vary. Most studies have shown that in families without peanut allergy, introducing peanuts to the diet at an early age reduces risk of later allergy. Some countries that tend to introduce peanuts early have lower peanut allergy rates than those that delay peanuts. Women who eat peanuts during pregnancy and breastfeeding reduce the rate of peanut allergy in their children. Our general advice at this time is to introduce peanut butter to infants between nine and twelve months of age; we see no need to delay longer than that.

What if peanut allergy runs in the family? Allergic parents may be hesitant to allow peanuts into their children's diet. Unfortunately, research hasn't provided a clear answer on whether or not such children should remain peanut-free in the early years. If a mother has peanut allergy, she is obviously not going to eat peanuts during pregnancy and breastfeeding, but perhaps she should carefully allow peanut butter between nine and twelve months with the approval of the doctor. If only Dad is allergic, then Mom should *not* avoid peanuts during pregnancy and breastfeeding, as research indicates that peanuts in Mom's diet may prevent the allergy in her children, despite Dad's genetics.

How careful do I have to be around peanuts? This varies depending on each individual's history of reactions. Not everyone who tests allergic or has a history of allergic reaction needs to live in a 100 percent peanut-sterile environment. It may be that your child can be around others who are eating peanut products. Some people, on the other hand, have allergic reactions simply from smelling peanuts or breathing in the odor from an opened peanut container in the same room, although anaphylactic reactions in such situations are rare. Theoretically, 100 percent avoidance of anything peanut should help you outgrow the allergy; however, research suggests that periodic exposures to small quantities of allergens may in fact help you eventually become *less* sensitive. That's the logic behind desensitization therapy. You will learn over time how careful you have to be, and your doctor will counsel you in this matter.

TREE NUT ALLERGY

Tree nuts include walnuts, pecans, almonds, cashews, pistachios, hazelnuts, chestnuts, macadamia nuts, and Brazil nuts. Peanuts, as you read above, are not tree nuts but legumes. However, practically speaking, much of the information written for peanut allergy (severity of reactions, diagnostic testing, and hidden foods to avoid) is virtually identical for tree nuts. Between 25 and 50 percent of peanut-allergic people will also have an allergy to at least one tree nut. The prognosis for outgrowing tree nut allergy is slightly worse at only about 10 percent. Tree nut allergy among children has increased even faster than peanut allergy; a fivefold increase since the mid-1990s now puts tree nut allergy at about 1 percent of children.

Common Questions

Is coconut a tree nut? No, coconut is a fruit and can be eaten by those with nut allergy. Also, to clarify, nutmeg, butternut squash, and water chestnuts are not nuts. Pine nuts are considered seeds, not nuts.

If a person is allergic to one tree nut, can he or she eat other tree nuts? Opinions vary on this. Many people test allergic to multiple tree nuts and simply avoid them all. Some with only one positive test may carefully try other nuts and consume them as tolerated. An allergist will provide you with guidance specific to your situation.

If I have a tree nut allergy, can I eat peanuts? The answer is probably yes. Your doctor will likely have tested you for peanut allergy while evaluating the tree nut allergy, and those test results will help answer this question. You should follow the same food avoidance guidelines listed under "hiding places" of peanuts above, but you can enjoy uncontaminated peanut products with your doctor's approval, as long as you verify that the product was not cross-contaminated with tree nuts during manufacturing.

POLLEN AND FOOD CROSS-REACTIVITY

An interesting syndrome exists in which people who are allergic to ragweed, birch pollen, or grass will feel mild allergic symptoms (itching and swelling) of the lips, mouth, or throat when they eat some of the following foods *raw:* apples, bananas, carrots, celery, cherries, cucumbers, hazelnuts, kiwifruit, melons, oranges, peaches, peanuts, pears, plums, potatoes, soy, tomatoes, and zucchini. These people aren't directly allergic to these foods, and food allergy testing will often be normal for them. Instead, they are allergic to the pollen, but their IgE antibodies cross-react with these foods when they are consumed raw. This phenomenon is called oral allergy syndrome, or pollen-associated food allergy syndrome. Fortunately, the reactions are minor and brief, and these foods need not be avoided unless they prove bothersome.

FISH AND SHELLFISH ALLERGY

These two allergies may seem similar on first glance, but there are significant distinctions. Some people are allergic to both fish and shellfish, but more often a person is allergic to only one and can safely enjoy the other.

Fish Allergy

Those who are allergic to fish are sometimes allergic to *all* fish. However, as fish are a very important and healthy part of the diet, consultation with an allergist and a determination of which fish may be safe are warranted. Testing for some specific types of fish is available (codfish, salmon, and tuna, for example) to help you determine how broad the allergy is, but many fish don't have a specific test yet. Your doctor will advise you on how to explore potential nonallergenic fish. Those with a fish allergy may outgrow it, but most will not.

Shellfish Allergy

Shellfish allergy is a much greater problem than fish allergy. It is more common, and it causes a greater severity of anaphylaxis than most other allergies. Shellfish allergy is rare in children; it generally develops during adulthood and is lifelong in virtually all sufferers. Those who are allergic to one shellfish are generally allergic to all. There are two types of shellfish:

Crustaceans. These include crab, lobster, and shrimp. Severe allergy to these is more common than severe allergy to the mollusks (below). Each crustacean can be tested separately, but in practice those who are allergic to one crustacean are generally advised to avoid all.

Mollusks. Clams, oysters, scallops, and mussels are the mollusks that are primarily responsible for allergy. Octopus, squid, and snails are also mollusks, but allergy to these is usually independent of the primary mollusks. Specific allergy tests are available for some mollusks.

Hidden Sources of Fish and Shellfish

Here are some specific foods and situations to be aware of:

Seafood restaurants. If your allergy is severe, it may be nearly impossible to avoid cross-contamination in a restaurant that is dedicated to seafood. Avoid fish markets as well. When you do go to a nonseafood restaurant, be sure the staff is aware of your allergy. Fish and shellfish proteins may rise into the air during cooking, and those who are severely allergic should avoid close proximity.

Food labels. Labeling on foods is very clear if shellfish (especially the crustaceans) is involved. Fish and shellfish are rarely hidden in unsuspected foods, although there are a few surprising places where fish may be found: Worcestershire sauce, Caesar salad dressing, and imitation crab (which is actually fish). Fish stock, often used in Asian cuisine, may contain shellfish as well.

EGG ALLERGY

Egg allergy is a particular challenge because eggs are so widely used in baking and are a staple of the American breakfast. On the other hand, eggs are less likely to trigger anaphylaxis in those who are allergic. Instead, egg reactions tend to present themselves on the skin. Egg allergy usually begins at an early age; for infants and young children with eczema or hives, you and your doctor should rule out egg allergy (along with milk and wheat) as a possible cause. Most people (75 percent) with egg allergy will outgrow it by adulthood.

There is currently no mainstream desensitization therapy for egg allergy, as there is for peanut allergy. However, researchers have studied the process, and the results look promising. Allergists will likely begin offering this option in the coming years. In addition, most people with egg allergy are allergic to the egg white but not the yolk, and most allergy tests only measure egg white protein allergy. Such people may be able to enjoy egg yolk, with permission from their doctor, if no allergy symptoms are seen. Following are some details that are unique to egg allergy.

Hidden Sources of Egg

Here are some not-so-obvious foods that may leave egg, and a rash, on your face:

- Almost all baked goods (egg-free recipes are available online)
- Some meat loaf and meatballs

- Some cream fillings and custard
- Breakfast casseroles
- Canned soup
- Salad dressing
- Ice cream
- Egg substitutes (these often contain egg whites)
- Mayonnaise
- Some marshmallow recipes (usually not store-bought)
- Meringue
- Nougat
- Some noodles
- Shiny glaze on baked goods

Component Allergy Blood Test

Similar to the test for peanut and milk allergies, ImmunoCAP offers this blood test for eggs. It measures allergy to ovalbumin, a protein that is broken down easily by heat; those who are primarily allergic to this protein may be able to tolerate cooked egg and are likely to outgrow the allergy. Ovomucoid is a second protein that is tested, and this one doesn't break down with heat; allergy to this protein warrants complete elimination of both cooked and raw egg, and people with this allergy are less likely to outgrow it.

Egg Allergy and Vaccines

Two routine childhood vaccines contain egg products. The MMR vaccine contains traces of chick embryo proteins left over from when the viruses are grown in the manufacturing process. This minute amount is unlikely to trigger an allergic reaction, and it is okay to get the MMR vaccine if you are egg-allergic.

The flu vaccine, however, is a different story. All flu viruses are grown in eggs, and a considerable amount of egg protein is left over in the final vaccine solution. The mainstream medical position on this issue holds that the risk of allergic reaction is small, and the importance of the flu vaccine is great; therefore, those who are allergic to eggs should still be vaccinated, and medical personnel should be ready to provide help if an allergic reaction occurs. In our office, we generally don't give flu vaccine to egg-allergic patients unless the person is a strong candidate for the vaccine, suffering from an underlying heart condition, asthma, or immune deficiency. In such people, the benefit of the flu vaccine may be higher than the small risk of allergic reaction. Those who are healthy and don't have an underlying medical condition, but who are allergic to eggs, may not want to risk the vaccine. Discuss this with your doctor.

SOY ALLERGY

This seemingly healthy food has come under fire in the past decade for several reasons. First, its estrogen-like properties have many health experts advising that we limit our intake. Second, almost all soy used in the United States is genetically modified (GMO), which may make it more allergenic. Soy is also in the same legume family as peanuts; the two share similar protein structures, and there is considerable allergenic cross-reactivity between them. But perhaps the most significant impact soy has on our nation's allergies comes from the fact that soy is now everywhere. If soy was only in soy sauce, tofu, and veggie burgers, many of us would only have occasional exposure. Instead, soy's allergenic properties infuse many of our daily foods and products; soy is an additive in most processed foods and is used in many vitamin supplements and nonfood products (as soy lecithin). Some experts propose that this almost daily exposure to GMO soy has contributed to the overall rise in allergic disorders; Robyn O'Brien discusses the GMO soy controversy in more detail, along with that of peanut and corn, in her book, *The Unhealthy Truth*.

The one saving grace about soy allergy is that most people

who are allergic are only mildly so, with anaphylaxis being extremely rare. Most reactions manifest as allergic skin rashes or as mood and behavioral problems. So the good news is that soy allergy won't kill you. But if you are sensitive or allergic and don't know it, daily GMO soy exposure can contribute to your long-term problems. Most kids will outgrow soy allergy (approximately 70 percent by age ten), and many will also lose their soy sensitivity over time. Below is what you need to know about soy.

Hidden Sources of Soy

Soy is rarely hidden. It is easy to find on any list of ingredients as soy, hydrolyzed soy protein, soybean, or soy lecithin. Here are some common sources that may be less obvious:

- Vegetable oils
- Margarine
- Mayonnaise
- Chocolate and chocolate desserts
- Baked goods
- Some canned tuna
- Processed meats
- Some deli meats
- Hot dogs
- Chicken nuggets
- Soups
- Sauces
- Meat substitutes
- Sausages
- Smoothie powders
- Commercial seasoning mixes
- Edamame
- Energy and nutrition bars
- Some nut butters and low-fat peanut butter
- Textured vegetable protein
- Nondairy creamer
- Many vitamins and nutritional supplements
- Most Asian cuisine contains soy, labeled in the following ways: kyodofu, miso, natto, okara, shoyu, soya, supro, tamari, tempeh, teriyaki, yakidofu, and yuba

Behavioral Versus Allergic Reactions

Those who have classic allergic reactions to soy may be able to handle some forms of soy without consequence; soy lecithin and highly refined soybean oil may be tolerated. Children with *behavioral* sensitivity to soy, on the other hand, may not be able to handle any exposure at all. In addition, many who are behaviorally sensitive to milk are also sensitive to soy. Finally, much of soy's reactivity may come from its genetic modification; organic, non-GMO soy may be okay. Experience will help you sort out these variations.

Soy Estrogen Controversy

The debate continues over whether soy is okay to eat even if we are not sensitive or allergic, with no clear answer just yet. Some health experts believe that eating fermented soy foods is the healthiest way to consume soy. These include tempeh, miso, natto, and traditionally made fermented soy sauce. Someday, research will provide definitive answers to the soy dilemma. For now, just as in most areas of life, the best advice is to enjoy it in moderation.

CORN ALLERGY

Corn is not found on most lists of common allergenic foods. That's because traditionally these lists present the top eight allergy foods. But if number nine were included, it would be corn. Corn shares two of soy's concerns: most of it is genetically modified, and it is used in many American foods in the form of

(continued)

corn syrup. Ironically, hypoallergenic infant formulas (used for those who are allergic to milk-based formula) are sweetened with corn syrup. Corn allergy is an increasing challenge for a growing number of Americans; those with food allergy symptoms should consider this as a possible culprit. Corn can also trigger behavioral problems in children, and those who try a milk-free, gluten-free, and soy-free diet without improvement should consider removing corn and corn syrup. One of the Sears children was very behaviorally sensitive to corn syrup growing up, and we see this on occasion in our practice.

FOOD ADDITIVE AND PRESERVATIVE ALLERGY AND SENSITIVITY

Finally, we wrap up our food allergy discussion with a reminder about the various chemicals that are used in our modern-day food industry. Gone are the days when local farmers carted their meat, eggs, milk, and produce to sell in the town square and bakers rose early every morning to prepare the daily bread for the townsfolk. Our expanded modern society necessitates that food be preserved so that it can be safely distributed and sold. That's a given. But what is completely *un*necessary is what we've done to our food: artificial colors, flavors, and sweeteners, plus insecticides and other chemicals, have become a part of the modern human food chain. For some reason, food makers believe our food must be bright and colorful, supersweet, and full of extra flavor. Maybe that's because such foods sell and healthy foods don't. Or because healthy foods cost more, so people are more likely to buy the cheaper stuff. And many of us are teaching our children bad lessons with the products we purchase: cereal Os have to be colorful, snacks must be sweet and come in a convenient package, and every meal must be wrapped in white bread (or maybe a light brown "whole grain" color). And heaven forbid that we actually snack on a piece of whole fruit!

If you or someone in your family is suffering from chronic allergies or behavioral problems, it's time to clean things up. Chemicals harm the immune system, cause inflammation, and can make allergic disorders worse. Classic allergic reactions to food chemicals are fairly rare, but they do occur. Behavioral reactions, on the other hand, are fairly common. Testing for allergy or sensitivity to chemicals is not considered accurate; instead, diet restriction followed by reintroduction is the standard way to diagnose a chemical allergy or sensitivity. Even if you are healthy, the changes discussed in this section will do you some good.

Interestingly, some naturally occurring chemicals are present in high levels in some natural foods. These are oxalates, phenols, and salicylates. These substances are harmless to most of us, but some people still have behavioral sensitivities to them. These are presented in detail at the end of this chapter.

Most Common Chemical Allergies and Sensitivities

Here are the most likely chemical culprits that may be responsible for behavioral food sensitivities and, in some cases, allergies:

Monosodium glutamate. MSG is used as a flavor enhancer in many soups, broths, gravies, flavored foods, powdered food mixes, imitation meats, sauces, and marinades. It is suspected of causing headaches, neurological symptoms, hyperactivity, attention difficulty, intestinal problems, and many other symptoms. However, some research studies have failed to show that MSG is a definite cause of harmful symptoms when consumed in low to moderate quantities.

The ingredient in MSG that is most concerning is glutamate. Glutamate is an amino acid, and it is a healthy and essential part of our body's metabolism. The worry is not glutamate itself;

rather, it is the quantity of added glutamate to which some people react. In large doses, this amino acid causes a rush of brain hormones that triggers uncomfortable neurological or body symptoms. The key to avoiding this reaction is to avoid large doses of artificially added glutamate in any shape, whether it's MSG or another form. Here are some of the hidden sources of glutamate in food:

- Hydrolyzed vegetable protein
- Autolyzed yeast
- Hydrolyzed yeast
- Yeast extract
- Protein isolate
- Glutamate or glutamic acid
- Certain processed proteins (whey, soy, caseinate, textured)
- Modified enzymes

Artificial food coloring. Of all the chemicals that can trigger behavioral problems, this tops the list. Any color followed by a number (such as Red Dye #40) can cause a problem. Every behavioral consultation we provide in our office begins with the recommendation to take out all artificial colors. True allergic reactions are extremely rare.

Artificial flavors. These chemicals are derived from a variety of unusual animal organs, petroleum, or coal tar. You will generally find them labeled as something like *artificial cherry flavor,* for example. Vanillin, a commonly used artificial vanilla flavor, however, does not require the label *artificial.* Allergic reactions are rare, but behavioral sensitivities are not.

Artificial preservatives. These can cause behavioral reactions as well as allergy symptoms. Sulfites, in particular, are known to trigger wheezing in many asthmatics. Health food manufacturers have turned to more natural ingredients to preserve food, but conventional food makers still use the following artificial preservatives, which you can look for on the label:

- BHA
- BHT
- TBHQ
- Nitrates/nitrites
- Sulfates/sulfites
- Benzoate

Artificial sweeteners. These rarely cause allergic reactions, but they can affect behavior. Here are the "bad" words to look for:

- Aspartame (NutraSweet, Equal)
- Saccharin (Sweet'N Low)
- Sucralose (Splenda; may be preferred over the first two)
- Corn syrup (although this is not an artificial sweetener, some people are corn-sensitive)
- High-fructose corn syrup (also not artificial, but it has gotten a bad rap for its possible negative effects on blood sugar and insulin balance)

The two healthiest natural substitute sugars are stevia, made from the plant of the same name, and xylitol, made from birch tree bark (though some xylitol is made from corn). Evaporated cane juice is another common, and safe, replacement. In moderation, plain white sugar may be safer than the artificial sugars.

Pesticides. Residual pesticides on foods don't cause direct allergic reactions, but their effect on the hormonal systems of the body can contribute to chronic allergic disorders. They rarely cause noticeable behavioral reactions like hyperactivity or aggression. However, they are neurotoxic, meaning they kill brain cells. So ultimately they can affect the development and function of the brain. It's best to steer clear of pesticides whenever you can. If you can't afford to go completely organic, here are the most pesticide-laden foods that you and your family should avoid:

- Apples
- Celery
- Cherry tomatoes
- Cucumbers
- Grapes
- Hot peppers
- Imported nectarines

- Kale and collard greens
- Peaches
- Potatoes
- Spinach
- Strawberries
- Summer squash
- Sweet bell peppers

This list, called the Dirty Dozen Plus, was determined by the Environmental Working Group and is updated periodically on its website, EWG.org.

PAINT YOUR HOUSE GREEN

Not literally. But you should realize that chemicals don't just come from food. They are present in many of the products we use in our daily lives, including our dishes, bottles, toys, cosmetics, furniture, personal hygiene products, clothes, household cleaners, and many other items. Plastics and flame retardants are among the worst offenders upon our immune and neurologic systems. You should try to make your family home as green as possible by limiting chemical exposure. You will find many useful life-cleaning guides on EWG.org.

Phenols and salicylates. These are two naturally occurring food-based chemicals that can irritate the nervous system and trigger behavioral problems. They also appear as artificial additives in some foods. Symptoms of sensitivity include hyperactivity, aggression, irritability, red cheeks, red ears, sleep problems, and bedwetting (or daytime accidents). These can also cause classic allergy signs like eczema and hives, although these are less common. Dr. Benjamin Feingold originally developed the idea of restricting these two chemicals in the diet (he proposed the Feingold diet in 1973) as a way to alleviate allergic diseases and behavioral disorders, and there is some research to back up his theory. A complete discussion on phenol and salicylate elimination can be found on Dr. Feingold's website and in his books, as well as on other websites that have built on his ideas. There is no accurate way to predict or test whether a particular person is sensitive. Suspect this problem in children with the above symptoms who have normal allergy test results. Any child or adult with chronic mood or behavioral problems may benefit from a trial of eliminating the following foods:

- Almost all of the artificial additives, preservatives, colors, and flavors listed in the preceding sections; they are all high in phenols, and eliminating them is the first and most important step in the Feingold program
- Fruits: apples, apricots, grapes, raisins, peaches, nectarines, oranges, plums, prunes, and pineapples
- Vegetables: bell peppers, chili peppers, tomatoes, pickles, and cucumbers
- Most berries
- Almonds
- Coffee, tea, and colas
- Honey
- Most spices: cayenne, chili powder, cinnamon, cumin, curry, dill, mustard, oregano, paprika, pepper, rosemary, sage, tarragon, turmeric, and thyme

Most of these foods are very healthy; it is important to try this elimination diet independently of any other new treatment or dietary trial so that you can accurately assess whether it is worth depriving your body of these nutritious foods. First eliminate the artificial foods and observe if improvements are significant without reducing the natural food phenols and salicylates just yet. Then reduce the food sources and see if further benefits are worth reducing these healthy foods. These chemicals can be addictive; if your child loves to smother everything in ketchup or tomato sauce, that might be a sign of abnormal cravings for these sensitive foods. If you are certain that this diet helps, read further online for more detailed lists of foods that can be eliminated. You won't have to follow this diet forever; as your body heals, you can learn what is tolerable in the years to come.

Oxalates. Oxalates are another naturally occurring chemical component in many healthy foods. In small amounts, they are harmless. Our healthy intestinal bacteria process oxalates so they pass harmlessly out through the stools. Yet those with imbalanced intestinal flora, and those with inflamed, leaky guts may absorb too many oxalates, which can then disperse into the bloodstream and crystallize in any body tissues that are already inflamed, causing pain and further inflammation in those tissues. This can manifest itself as hyperactivity, severe tantrums, out-of-control behavior, or neurodevelopmental delays. They can also cause kidney stones.

Oxalate sensitivity is an emerging theory in the area of behavioral reactions to food. There is a growing body of research that shows it can cause food-related behavioral problems, yet not enough for it to become an accepted idea just yet. Oxalate levels can be measured in the urine through most laboratories, but high levels in the urine aren't a guarantee that the crystals are actually causing any internal problems. The only treatment approach so far is to limit the amount of high-oxalate foods in the diet. Foods that are highest in oxalates include:

- Soy and beans (black, kidney, navy, pinto)
- Wheat and rye
- Carrots, canned tomato sauce and paste, olives, potatoes, sweet potatoes, and spinach
- Oranges
- Chocolate and tea
- Tree nuts (almonds, cashews, hazelnuts, walnuts), peanuts, and sesame seeds

Eliminating, or at least limiting, these foods for a few months should result in behavioral improvements if oxalates are a problem. Reduce the foods gradually over two months; sudden removal of all foods can draw too much oxalate out of body tissues into the bloodstream and cause worsened symptoms. If you do conclude that there is improvement, you should explore more detailed lists of oxalate foods online to make sure you are eliminating them properly. The most thorough online resource is LowOxalate.info.

An additional solution is to heal the leaky gut and restore intestinal bacteria. We agree. Oxalate food restriction may be valuable for short-term behavioral benefits, but it shouldn't be necessary in the long run. Chapter 14 describes how to heal the leaky gut and reduce body inflammation for better long-term health.

Move to an Organic Farm

When counseling patients with food-related behavioral challenges, we jokingly advise them to move to an organic farm. But more seriously, we strongly advise these families to buy and eat food *as if* they live on an organic farm. This means you should buy almost nothing that comes packaged for mass production or has a long shelf life. All produce, dairy products, berries, nuts, and eggs that you eat should be organic. Meats should be grass-fed and organic. Foods should be whole and fresh, not processed into artificial shapes. Veggies should actually be veggies, not puff snacks. Transform your family's food as thoroughly as your situation warrants; the more severe your family's food sensitivities, the greater the transformation.

10

Other Food Allergy and Sensitivity Syndromes (EoE, FPIES, Histamine Intolerance, GERD, Fructose Malabsorption, and Colic)

In addition to the straightforward food allergies discussed in the preceding chapters, three newly discovered food sensitivity syndromes affect a growing number of children but are not well known. These are eosinophilic gastrointestinal disorders (eosinophilic esophagitis [EoE or EE], gastritis, colitis, and gastroenteritis), food protein–induced enterocolitis syndrome (FPIES), and histamine intolerance. Gastroesophageal reflux disease (GERD) is also a food-sensitivity syndrome, as is fructose malabsorption and infant colic. This chapter offers a brief discussion of each and gets you started on the road to diagnosis and treatment.

EOSINOPHILIC GASTROINTESTINAL DISORDERS

These are a group of allergic disorders that have only recently been recognized in the world of medicine. Instead of the usual IgE-mediated allergic response of mast cells and other immune cells described on page 8, the eosinophil class of immune cells plays a primary role in these disorders (eosinophils are one of the types of white blood cells responsible for allergic reactions—see page 5). The underlying mechanism is an allergic/inflammatory reaction to food (and possibly to pollen and other airborne allergens) that triggers the eosinophils in the lining of the gastrointestinal tract to release their allergen-fighting chemicals. These irritating chemicals cause painful burning in the area of the GI tract where they are released. Other cells, like lymphocytes and mast cells, are thought to be involved in this inflammatory process as well.

Four distinct eosinophilic GI conditions have been identified so far, and they are named according to the part of the GI tract that reacts: eosinophilic esophagitis, known as EoE or EE, occurs in the esophagus, or lower part of the throat; eosinophilic gastritis takes place in the stomach; eosinophilic colitis is confined to the colon; and eosinophilic gastroenteritis occurs throughout the entire GI tract. EoE is the first of these entities to be discovered and seems to be the most common, so our discussion will focus on this, with references to the rest of the GI tract.

Despite the fact that eosinophilic GI disorders are fairly new, specialists have a pretty accurate understanding of the causes and have worked out standard approaches to diagnosis, which we will explain below. However, doctors have not quite settled on the best therapies just yet. Several options are available that work very well, but we cannot yet say what the best therapy will be for you or your child. We present you with some options that you and your doctor will consider.

These disorders are tied closely to other allergic disorders. Research shows that about 80 percent of people with an eosinophilic GI disorder (especially EoE) have at least one other major allergic disorder (nasal allergies, asthma, eczema, and/or food allergy). Eosinophilic GI disorders also run in families (if one child has a disorder, many, if not most, of the remaining children will have it as well), and it can be passed genetically from parent to child.

Unfortunately, at this time it is thought that people do not outgrow eosinophilic GI disorders. Symptoms can be resolved by avoiding the offending allergens and using appropriate medications, but the problems eventually return when therapy and diet are stopped. The underlying allergic and inflammatory susceptibilities remain, and at this time they may be too genetically ingrained to eliminate completely.

Eosinophilic Esophagitis (EoE)

Eosinophilic esophagitis was recently discovered in groups of patients who were being evaluated for gastroesophageal reflux disease, or GERD. These children and adults were suffering from heartburn, but they were not responding well to heartburn medication. Further investigation with endoscopy and esophageal biopsies revealed high numbers of eosinophils, along with inflammatory changes, in the lining of the lower esophagus. Classically, patients with GERD have inflammation (from stomach acid burning the esophagus) but not many eosinophils. This discovery led GI and allergy specialists to realize that a new, allergy-based disorder was affecting this group, and thus EoE was named.

Cause. EoE is caused by food allergies. The eight most commonly allergic foods discussed in the preceding chapters are the most likely culprits. It is not known, however, why EoE sufferers have such a severe GI reaction to these foods compared to those who have only classic allergies; the additional allergic/inflammatory reaction in EoE is likely genetically mediated. Those with EoE also seem to experience worsened symptoms during times of high pollen counts; pollen is unlikely a primary cause but is a contributing factor nonetheless.

Symptoms. Symptoms vary with age. Infants and toddlers present with symptoms that mimic GERD: regurgitation or vomiting, feeding difficulties, irritability, and possibly failure to gain weight. School-age children will continue to have regurgitation or vomiting and will complain of significant abdominal pain. Over the years, however, the chronically inflamed esophagus becomes dysfunctional, and teens and adults will report difficulty swallowing, as well as heartburn and upper abdominal pain. Food may even become stuck as the esophagus narrows and hardens.

It is theorized that the inflammatory reaction to food in EoE is not immediate, as in most allergic reactions; rather, the allergenic foods cause a sustained and chronic inflammatory reaction in the lining of the esophagus, causing symptoms while eating as well as between meals.

It can be difficult to distinguish between EoE and GERD because the symptoms are so similar. A primary clue is that antacid medications generally resolve GERD symptoms. With EoE, they may reduce symptoms slightly, but not enough to bring lasting relief. Any person diagnosed with GERD who doesn't respond well to therapy should be evaluated for EoE. In addition, those with allergic disorders who also complain of GERD symptoms should be considered for evaluation.

Diagnosis. The gold standard of EoE diagnosis is to find a high number of eosinophils and inflammation on an esophageal biopsy during an upper endoscopy procedure. This can be confirmed by seeing resolution of the eosinophilic inflammation on subsequent endoscopic biopsies after therapy has begun.

Testing for allergies. The key to successful treatment is to determine which foods the person is allergic to. For EoE, it is currently thought that skin testing is more accurate than blood testing. In addition, food patch testing (placing a food directly on the skin for forty-eight hours and measuring the reaction) has particular usefulness in detecting EoE allergens.

Treatment options. At this time there is no cure for EoE. Specialists have developed several options for minimizing the immune system's response to the offending allergens through food avoidance and allergy treatments, but the underlying immune sensitivity to the allergenic foods remains:

> **Food avoidance based on allergy test results.** Those who show significant food allergies on blood, skin, and/or patch testing should strictly avoid those foods. For some sufferers, this will be enough to limit the inflammation.

> **Full elimination diet.** Some people must eliminate all eight of the most common food allergens (milk, wheat, eggs, soy, fish, shellfish, tree nuts, and peanuts). This allows the allergic part of the immune system to calm down, and the eosinophilic inflammation decreases.

> **Elemental formula diet.** In this more extreme approach, *all* food proteins are removed from the diet. Patients eat a formula made up of amino acids, carbohydrates, fats, vitamins, and minerals. This is a fairly practical approach for infants who are already on formula. For children and adults it is obviously far more challenging, as these age groups may not comply with such a limited diet for long.

> **Medications to reduce inflammation.** Oral steroids have been shown to improve symptoms in EoE patients, and appropriate courses under the close guidance of a physician can bring much-needed relief. The proton-pump inhibitor class of antacid medications (omeprazole and its newer versions) can also reduce esophageal inflammation (though other types of antacids don't seem to help).

> **Combination therapy.** Many EoE treatment centers are finding that a combination of diet restriction, steroid therapy, and antacid medication brings relief to most patients.

**SHOULD YOU CONSULT AN ALLERGIST OR
A GI SPECIALIST FOR EoE?**

Because EoE causes gastrointestinal symptoms, GI specialists
have been in the forefront of discovering and managing it. However, it has become apparent that EoE and the other eosinophilic
gastrointestinal syndromes are allergic and immunologic disorders. The current standard of care, therefore, is to consult with a
team of GI and allergy/immunology specialists who have joined
forces to provide care for patients with EoE. Most large university medical centers and children's hospitals now have such
teams. Ask your doctor for a referral to one near you. In the coming years, most individual GI and allergy/immunology specialists will likely begin caring for these patients as standard
treatments are developed.

Eosinophilic Gastroenteritis (EG) and Colitis (EC)

These two conditions are far less common than EoE. Problems
usually occur more in the lower GI tract, with abdominal pain,
diarrhea, nausea, vomiting, and weight loss as the primary symptoms. Those with EG may also have some difficulty in swallowing, as with EoE and GERD. The diagnosis is made through
endoscopy. Treatment approaches are similar to those for EoE.
EC seems to respond particularly well to the removal of cow's
milk and soy from the diet.

FOOD PROTEIN–INDUCED ENTEROCOLITIS SYNDROME (FPIES)

This is another newcomer to food sensitivity disorders, and it
affects less than 1 percent of infants. FPIES occurs due to an
immune sensitivity to certain food proteins.

Cause of FPIES

Instead of the classic IgE type of allergic reaction, researchers suspect it is the T lymphocytes that react to a small number of specific food proteins and trigger a delayed allergic reaction. Infants are likely born with a genetic susceptibility to FPIES, although we don't yet know which genes are responsible or how to predict who may be at risk.

Solid baby foods that have been found to trigger an FPIES reaction include (in order of commonness):

- Rice
- Oats
- Wheat
- Barley
- Sweet potatoes
- Bananas
- Poultry
- Peas
- Green beans
- Squash
- Fish
- Eggs

Cow's milk or soy infant formula can also trigger reactions; proteins passing through Mom's breast milk can very rarely cause FPIES reactions.

Symptoms of FPIES

FPIES has a classic and predictable pattern. Severe vomiting occurs about two hours after ingestion of the reactive food. It will seem as if the victim is experiencing food poisoning. Repetitive vomiting will persist for several hours, and diarrhea will usually set in. In many cases, symptoms will resolve without any treatment as the reaction runs its course.

Some cases, however, will progress into a shocklike state from a drop in blood pressure; the patient can become pale and lethargic and appear severely dehydrated. It's as if the person is having an anaphylactic reaction without the wheezing and without the classic skin signs of itching, hives, and swelling. Although fairly uncommon, such reactions require a trip to an emergency room for intravenous hydration and stabilization.

Diagnosing FPIES

Interestingly, food allergy tests are usually normal in these children and don't help identify the offending foods. Endoscopy is usually not necessary; when done, it will often reveal inflammation within the GI tract.

The diagnosis is primarily made by observing the pattern of the reactions. FPIES presents with the following unique features, which easily distinguish it from GERD (reflux), the stomach flu, or food poisoning:

It often begins between three and seven months of age but may begin at twelve months or later. Most infants are born healthy and have no feeding problems during the first few months. Then the first episode of intense vomiting suddenly occurs. GERD, on the other hand, usually begins within the first few weeks.

It is episodic. Repetitive vomiting occurs for several hours, then stops. After recovery, the infant may appear well for several days; then he or she has another episode. Spells will continue until a diagnosis is made. Food poisoning or stomach flu, which can be confused with FPIES, occurs only once every few months.

It predictably occurs about two hours after a feeding. GERD, or infant reflux, tends to occur right after a feeding, whereas the immune reaction in FPIES takes two to three hours to build up after a feeding.

It occurs after the first or second feeding of a suspect food. The first or second exposure to one of the above solid foods should provide a clue to the diagnosis. Some infants, on the other hand, will tolerate their infant formula in the early months, then begin to react to it. Previously healthy breastfed infants may suddenly react when Mom eats one of these foods, then breastfeeds the baby.

The vomiting is unusually intense. GERD usually involves milder regurgitation or, at the most, one or two vomits right after a feed; then the infant appears well. With FPIES, vomiting persists several times each hour for many hours, often followed by diarrhea. This pattern is somewhat indistinguishable from stomach flu or food poisoning at first; repeated episodes that become increasingly worse tell the tale.

Lethargy and shock may occur. Some infants, as described above, will experience a shocklike state from a drop in blood pressure. Repeated episodes that result in such emergencies should provide a clear clue to the diagnosis.

Emergency Care

Infants who are extremely pale or lethargic should receive emergency care. Intravenous fluids are usually needed, and, rarely, epinephrine may be given to assist in resuscitation in severe cases. Blood tests will likely be done to assess hydration status and check for infectious causes. Steroids may be useful in shortening the reaction.

Fortunately, most infants don't progress this far into the reaction; vomiting persists for several hours, then ends, and the infant recovers without any lasting effects.

Diagnostic Oral Food Challenge

Some experts advise that infants receive a test feeding of the reactive food in a controlled environment, such as an allergist's office, in order to observe the reaction and confirm the diagnosis. This is unnecessary if the infant's history is already obvious for FPIES. It may be useful if the diagnosis is in doubt.

Treating FPIES

The only known treatment at this time is avoidance of the reactive food. Most infants will react to only one or two foods, though some will react to the whole list. Breastfeeding moms will need to keep reactive foods out of the diet, and infants who react to a milk- or soy-based formula may need to use a hypoallergenic one (see formula choices on page 136). Your doctor will advise you whether to keep all FPIES foods out of your infant's diet, even those you haven't started yet, or to simply avoid the foods that cause a definite reaction.

Fortunately, children outgrow FPIES sensitivity by three or four years of age. You and your doctor will discuss how and when to carefully try these foods again.

HISTAMINE INTOLERANCE

This disorder occurs due to a deficiency of diamine oxidase, an intestinal enzyme that is necessary to break down naturally occurring histamines in food. When such foods are eaten, the large dose of histamine absorbs into the body and triggers symptoms of an allergic reaction. This is further complicated by a possible lack of another enzyme, histamine N-methyltransferase, which is supposed to deactivate histamine within the body. A detailed discussion of this rare disorder is beyond the scope of this book, but here are some key details to guide you.

Sufferers will experience recurrent, unexplained, seemingly allergic reactions to foods that range from mild symptoms to life-threatening anaphylactic shock. But the foods that trigger these reactions won't be the common allergens, and allergy testing will likely be normal because the patient isn't having a typical allergic reaction to the food proteins.

Diagnosis is made by strictly avoiding histamine foods for two to four weeks and observing resolution of histamine-induced symptoms. In research settings, blood tests for histamine enzymes can be done, but these aren't widely available to the public at this time. Ongoing food avoidance is currently the only known treatment. Antihistamine medications may be useful as well.

Here is a list of foods that may contain a high level of histamine:

- Spinach, eggplant, pumpkins, and tomatoes
- Citrus fruits, raisins, and fruits with pits (apricots, peaches, prunes, dates, and cherries)
- Nonfresh fish and shellfish, processed and smoked meats, eggs, walnuts, cashews, and peanuts
- Chocolate, tea, and artificial additives and preservatives
- Fermented foods (aged cheeses, beer, wine, sauerkraut, pickles, vinegar, soy sauce, tofu, miso, and tempeh)

Research and debate continue to yield more consensus on this newly recognized problem. Consultation with an allergy specialist will offer the most up-to-date guidance. The bottom line is to consider this condition if recurrent food-related allergic reactions persist despite thorough classic food allergy testing and treatment.

GASTROESOPHAGEAL REFLUX DISEASE (GERD)

GERD, or reflux, is not classically thought of as an allergic disorder. But because it is so common, and because it can be caused by food sensitivity, it deserves a brief mention. On page 110 we described how infant formula intolerance can present as reflux, as can sensitivity to foods passing through Mom's breast milk. In our opinion, reflux should be considered a food intolerance until proven otherwise. Here is how we approach this in our office:

Diagnosing Reflux

GERD is diagnosed by observing the pattern of spitting up. Diagnostic tests are rarely necessary. Classic symptoms include the following:

Spitting up after feeds. This is the primary symptom. The baby will regurgitate after some or most feeds; sometimes the baby will vomit up what seems like the entire feed.

Pain. Stomach acid that comes up with the regurgitated milk can burn the esophagus, causing painful, colicky fussing in infants.

Symptoms when lying flat. Those with reflux usually have worsened symptoms while lying flat on their back. This position more easily allows stomach acid to flow into the esophagus. Keeping a baby propped upright after feeds and during sleep can be used as a diagnostic trial to help confirm the suspected diagnosis.

Frequent night waking. Those with reflux tend to wake up frequently, often in pain.

Symptoms of older children and adults. Older children and adults can more accurately describe reflux symptoms. The most obvious one is heartburn; this classic sign is the primary diagnostic clue to reflux. Other signs that can be attributed to reflux include asthma, chronic throat clearing, difficulty swallowing, and recurrent sinus problems.

Is It a "Disease" or Just a Laundry Problem?

Regurgitation that doesn't result in painful crying, frequent night waking, or other complications really isn't a disease. It's GER without the *D*. Spitting up is inconvenient and messy, but infants will outgrow it over time. If necessary, this mild reflux can be alleviated by following the steps outlined below.

Resolving Reflux in Breastfed Infants

Reflux can occur in a breastfeeding mother/infant pair for the following reasons:

Foremilk overload. The first several minutes of a feeding provide milk that is higher in sugar. Infants who have short feedings from both breasts may experience some digestive discomfort from this overload of milk sugar. Prolonged feedings from one breast may help.

Overactive letdown. Some moms release a rush of milk during the first minutes of a feed, which can overwhelm a baby, causing him to gulp extra air as he tries to keep up with the flow. Slowing down these feeds may help.

Cow's milk or wheat sensitivity. By far, the most common reason for reflux disease in breastfed babies is sensitivity to one or both of these foods in Mom's diet. Every mother/baby pair with reflux should commit to at least two months without one or both of these foods. Other foods on the common food allergy list may also contribute. Periodically eat these foods so baby gets some exposure to help him eventually become tolerant of them.

Fussy foods. These foods may be physically irritating to a baby and cause colic or reflux: caffeine, chocolate, gassy vegetables (broccoli, cauliflower, brussels sprouts, bell peppers, cabbage, onions), and even prenatal vitamins.

Solving Reflux in Formula-Fed Infants

Try the following steps:

Feed half as much, twice as often. Smaller, slower feeds are more easily digested and result in less reflux. Learn what volume and frequency of feeds are best tolerated by your baby.

Consider a change of formula. The best-tolerated formulas for babies with reflux are called hypoallergenic formulas; the milk components are predigested and the sugars are less irritating. However, these formulas are so processed and artificial that their nutritional value may not be ideal. The best substitute source of nutrition for a baby who is not breastfeeding is donated breast milk, either from a milk bank or from a trusted family member or friend. A second choice well tolerated by most sensitive babies is a homemade formula recipe that uses either pasteurized goat milk or raw cow's milk as its base. See page 136 for more details on formula options.

FRUCTOSE MALABSORPTION

This little-known digestive problem often goes undetected, yet is fairly easy to diagnose and resolve once it is realized. Sufferers lack the digestive enzyme necessary for the intestines to digest fructose (fruit sugar), similar to lactose intolerance described on page 133. The undigested fructose ferments into gas and causes bloating, pain, diarrhea (or constipation, or both), and flatulence. Symptoms are usually brought on by a high-fructose meal, but can also occur independent of a meal due to chronic irritation and imbalanced intestinal bacteria. This condition is diagnosed with a hydrogen breath test (page 133), but it can also be diagnosed by observing improvement with a low-fructose diet and confirmation of returning symptoms from a high-fructose meal. Suspect it when all other GI and allergy testing has been normal, and other measures haven't brought resolution.

Primary treatment involves restricting fructose foods in the diet. Such foods include most fruit juices, apples, pears, mangos, cherries, peaches, fruit concentrates, honey, corn syrup, high-fructose corn syrup, whole corn, wheat (and anything made with wheat flour), onions, garlic, asparagus, artichokes, leeks, and green beans. In addition to diet restriction, a digestive enzyme can be taken to help digest the sugars without suffering symptoms. This is only a brief introduction to this disorder. More detailed information can be obtained online and from your doctor.

COLIC

Colic is a complicated challenge for many young babies. Detailed discussions are provided in two other books in the Sears Parenting Library: *The Baby Book* and *The Portable Pediatrician*. Colic is not an allergic disorder, but it can be caused by food sensitivity through Mom's diet or by formula intolerance, just as in GERD. Following the advice in Chapter 6, "Food Allergies and Sensitivities: Overview of Symptoms and Testing" and in the reflux section above may result in relief for infants who have colic. Colic should be considered a cow's milk or wheat/gluten intolerance until proven otherwise.

One emerging suspect that may contribute to colicky symptoms and formula intolerance deserves special mention: transient lactase deficiency. Lact*ase* is the intestinal enzyme that digests milk sugar, or lact*ose*. Some infants are transiently deficient in this enzyme, and the undigested milk sugars are fermented into gas lower down in the digestive tract. This can irritate the colon and cause painful colicky symptoms. Infant lactase digestive enzyme drops are available over-the-counter and can be added to infant formula with each feed for several months and then discontinued around four months of age, when most infants will begin generating enough of their own lactase enzymes. Transient lactase deficiency can occur in breastfed babies as well, and drops can be added to breast milk to aid in digestion. Consult with your doctor for more specific guidance.

11

Anaphylaxis: From Mild Hives to Life-Threatening Allergic Reactions

Anaphylactic reaction is the most feared aspect of allergic disorders. Fortunately, less than 1 percent of our population has an allergy severe enough to cause anaphylaxis, and when a severe reaction does occur, only about 1 percent will progress to fatality. Still, approximately 1,000 Americans die every year from a severe allergic reaction; most of these are from a medication allergy, and some are due to a reaction to food or an insect sting. The good news is that once an anaphylactic tendency is identified, measures can be taken to prevent further exposure, and patients can be prepared with a self-administered injection of epinephrine in case of emergency. This chapter contains what you need to know about diagnosing and managing anaphylaxis.

Far more common are mild allergic reactions that manifest as simple hives and other skin signs. While these are not considered true anaphylaxis, their causes and the approaches to treatment and prevention are similar. Therefore, we include a discussion of the evaluation and treatment of hives in this chapter.

IMMUNOLOGY OF HIVES AND ANAPHYLACTIC REACTIONS

This reaction begins like all of the others (review page 8). An allergen is introduced into a body tissue and binds to its specific IgE antibodies on the tissue mast cells, which release their cascade of chemicals (histamine, enzymes, nitric oxide, and cytokines) that initiate the allergic reaction. Basophils in the bloodstream also respond to the IgE and spread the allergic reaction to the rest of the body. The chemicals released by these immune cells cause the following reactions, which, when put together, result in anaphylaxis:

Blood vessels dilate. This not only brings more blood and reactive immune cells to the initial site of reaction, but it also helps spread the reaction to other body tissues. And when the blood vessels dilate too much, blood pressure drops and the victim goes into shock. The term *anaphylactic shock* refers to this response.

Blood vessels start to leak. Blood vessels become more leaky, or permeable, and allow fluids from the bloodstream to leak into body tissues. This causes swelling and draws even more irritating immune chemicals into the tissues. Victims will see the swelling anywhere on the body (most commonly the feet, hands, and face), and may feel the swelling in the mouth and throat. In the skin layers, this swelling manifests itself as hives.

Blood vessel and lung muscles constrict. Muscles that surround the blood vessels tighten up, which actually helps counteract blood vessel dilation and preserve blood pressure. But the muscles that surround the airways in the lungs and throat also contract, causing the victim to wheeze and have difficulty drawing in air.

Nerves are activated. Histamine also activates nerves in the affected area, which release a neurochemical that dilates blood vessels, constricts airways, and triggers even more histamine release into body tissues.

What factors determine whether an allergic response continues to the point of anaphylaxis or stops short somewhere along the way with only a mild to moderate allergic reaction? This is not yet well understood. We know that those with chronic asthma and a long history of other allergies (especially eczema) have much higher levels of IgE antibodies and reactive immune cells, and that such people are more prone to anaphylaxis. So it may be the sheer quantity of reactive immune cells and antibodies that causes someone to progress down this pathway. But there are other factors that we don't yet understand; for example, those who live closer to either pole of the earth are more likely to experience anaphylaxis, as are teenage girls. Fortunately, of the million or so anaphylactic reactions that occur each year in the United States, fewer than 1 percent are fatal.

SYMPTOMS AND TIMING OF ANAPHYLAXIS

Anaphylaxis can present with many different symptoms in various areas of the body, and some reactions may cause only one or two obvious signs. Classically, for an allergic reaction to be considered anaphylactic, two or more body systems need to be affected. But in practical terms, anyone with a severe, life-threatening episode with only one reactive body system would be diagnosed with anaphylaxis. Here are the signs of anaphylaxis, listed from the most common to the least common:

Skin Signs

Most people who are having an anaphylactic reaction (90 percent or more) will experience hives, swelling, flushing, and itching.

This may occur in only one area or may spread throughout the body. A common misconception is that when hives spread toward the neck, breathing difficulty will soon follow. This is not the case; location of hives does not correlate with severity of reaction.

Many allergic reactions will cause only hives and other skin signs and won't progress further. Although these are not considered true anaphylaxis, subsequent episodes have the potential to worsen. Causes should be identified, and treatment options should be made readily available (see the sections later in this chapter on treatment and prevention, pages 235 and 238).

Respiratory Signs

Only about 50 percent of people will experience wheezing, shortness of breath, or feelings of airway obstruction during anaphylaxis, and the presence of these signs increases the risk of fatality. Runny nose is also a respiratory manifestation, although a minor one. Some sufferers, especially those known to be asthmatic, may experience a sudden onset of respiratory difficulty without any preceding warning signs on the skin.

Cardiovascular Signs

Dizziness, fainting, chest pain, arrhythmia, or low blood pressure occurs in only one-third of adult sufferers, and less often in children. Outright heart attack is a rare, yet possible, cardiac complication. Only very rarely will a person go into sudden cardiac shock without any skin or respiratory warning signs.

Gastrointestinal Signs

Another one-third of people will experience nausea, vomiting, pain, or diarrhea, especially when the allergen has been ingested.

Timing of Signs

Timing and duration of symptoms vary greatly among individuals. Here are some common patterns to expect:

Onset of symptoms. Injected antigens (such as antibiotic shots or bee stings) tend to cause the fastest reactions; symptoms begin as quickly as within five minutes, or may be delayed for thirty minutes or more. Antigens that are swallowed often take longer but will usually cause a reaction within two hours. The more sudden the onset, the more likely the reaction is to progress to full anaphylaxis.

Duration of symptoms. Most reactions subside within one to two hours; the histamine and other immune chemicals are used up, and symptoms gradually go away. Rarely, anaphylactic reactions can persist for days. Reactions that are limited to hives can also persist for days, even weeks, especially when triggered by viral infections (see below).

Relapse of symptoms. A small percentage of sufferers will experience a relapse of symptoms eight to twenty-four hours after the initial reaction subsides; this is more common with food reactions and in those who experience shock (low blood pressure) during the initial reaction.

CAUSES OF HIVES AND ANAPHYLAXIS

Once you or your child has experienced an anaphylactic reaction, identifying the cause of the reaction is critical for future prevention. Here are the possible causes you and your doctor will consider:

No Cause

The majority of cases of severe allergic reactions don't have an identifiable cause. This is especially true for adults: no obvious food, medication, or insect culprit can be determined, and allergy test results may be normal. In children, an allergic cause for anaphylactic reactions is more often found, but sometimes can remain a mystery. We have sat with many patients over the years, wracking our brains to sort out the trigger, only to come up empty-handed.

Infection

Although rarely a cause in adults, infections may be the most common cause of hives in children (full anaphylaxis is virtually unheard of in infectious cases). When hives accompany or follow a fever or other signs of illness, pediatricians (ourselves included) will generally attribute the hives to the illness and not perform any allergy testing. Such hives can persist for weeks after the illness resolves. The most common infectious cause of hives is a variety of harmless viruses, which don't require specific diagnosis or treatment. Some bacterial infections, particularly one called mycoplasma, can trigger hives, as can some parasites and fungi. Your doctor will consider these based on your symptoms and physical findings.

Food

Food is the most commonly identified allergic cause. Chapters 6 through 10 discuss specific food allergies in detail. The most likely foods will vary depending on age.

The most common allergic foods in children are:

- Milk
- Eggs
- Peanuts

- Wheat
- Soy
- Tree nuts
- Fish

In adults, the most likely offenders are:

- Peanuts
- Tree nuts
- Fish
- Shellfish

Medications

These are a close second, especially in adults. The most likely causes are:

- Antibiotics
- Aspirin and other anti-inflammatory medications, like ibuprofen
- Opiate pain relievers, like morphine
- Intravenous solutions used for radiology procedures

Uncommon Causes of Acute Hives and Anaphylactic Reactions

The following are uncommon triggers but are important to consider when you are attempting to identify a cause:

- Latex allergy (from repetitive use of latex gloves and equipment in medical settings)
- Insect stings (by wasps, bees, hornets, or fire ants)
- Exercise (a very rare condition in which exercise after the ingestion of an allergic food or medication will trigger anaphylaxis)

- Extreme temperatures (cold or heat)
- Food additives, like MSG
- Contact with plants or animals
- Physical triggers, like pressure

Chronic Hives (Without Anaphylaxis)

Most cases of acute hives resolve within days or weeks without consequence. Rarely, hives will continue to flare intermittently for months or even years. Finding an identifiable cause of chronic hives on allergy testing is unlikely, as most cases of chronic, recurrent hives are not caused by the usual allergic culprits. Allergy testing is nevertheless appropriate, in case an allergic and preventable cause can be found. Here are some of the uncommon nonallergic causes of nonanaphylactic hives that you and your doctor should consider:

Physical causes. Various physical factors can trigger hive reactions in the skin. These are diagnosed based on observation and experience. Treatment and prevention involve avoidance of the physical trigger and medications as needed. Causes include:

- Pressure (from scratching, rubbing, wearing tight clothing, prolonged pressure on a body part from sitting or standing, using hand tools, or even hand clapping; can cause immediate or delayed swelling and/or hives)
- Heat (hot baths, exercise, or sweat)
- Anxiety (very rare)
- Cold temperatures (can be a familial trait)
- Sunlight (or sometimes certain indoor lights)
- Water (can trigger small, pinpoint hives)
- Vibrations (can trigger the swelling of an area, and sometimes hives)

Autoimmune disorders. Some autoimmune disorders, including thyroid disease, will present with chronic hives as one of the symptoms. Your doctor should consider these as a possible cause.

Chronic infections. Viruses such as Epstein-Barr, hepatitis, and herpes have been implicated as a possible cause, as have some parasites and fungi (like toenail or scalp infections). Testing for these may be warranted. Even chronic sinus infections may be a trigger. H. pylori (Helicobacter pylori, a stomach infection) has also been implicated.

Autoantibody-associated urticaria. This rare form of chronic hives occurs because a person's own IgG antibodies attack their own IgE antibodies on their immune cells within the skin. It isn't clear why this happens, but the result is a periodic hive reaction.

Testing for causes. In addition to allergy tests, a thorough medical history, physical exam, and medical testing may reveal a diagnosable and treatable cause of chronic hives. But in most cases, no such cause can be identified. Medication (see below) may be necessary to control symptoms.

TREATMENT OF HIVES AND ANAPHYLAXIS

A detailed discussion of emergency treatment for severe anaphylactic reactions is beyond the scope of this book. We will limit our information to what you can do to treat the initial phase of an allergic reaction, how to seek emergency care, and how to approach chronic hives.

Mild Reactions

If a reaction is mild, involving only hives and other skin signs, and the person is awake and alert, take the following measures:

Use antihistamine medication. Prompt treatment with diphenhydramine (commonly known by its brand name, Benadryl) will usually resolve the reaction within thirty minutes. This over-the-counter antihistamine comes in liquid, chewable, and tablet forms—just follow the suggested dosing on the package. For infants and toddlers who are too young for the package dosing instructions and for whom consultation with a doctor isn't immediately available, a dose of 1 milligram for every two pounds the child weighs is appropriate. For example, a 12.5-milligram dose would be given to a twenty-five-pound toddler (liquid and chewable forms are typically 12.5 milligrams per teaspoon or tablet). An infant who weighs about half that much would take half a dose. Commonly, hives will return as the medication wears off after six hours. Repeat the dose as needed if the reaction is uncomfortable; it is okay to allow mild hives to go untreated if a child isn't bothered by them.

Contact your doctor. Call your doctor's office to discuss whether or not your child should be seen that day. Most cases of hives will resolve with treatment and will eventually subside, even if not treated, as the histamine in the body runs out. If your child is alert and active and shows no other signs of anaphylaxis, an urgent appointment may not be necessary. If you suspect an obvious cause for the reaction (for example, your toddler just tried peanut butter for the first or second time), avoid that food until your next doctor's appointment. If a cause isn't apparent, see your doctor to discuss further diagnostic steps.

Anaphylactic Reactions

Sudden and severe allergic reactions are scary. Fortunately, fatalities are rare if prompt and proper emergency steps are followed:

Call 911. As soon as you realize that an anaphylactic reaction is beginning (whether it is in yourself or someone else), call 911 so that emergency personnel will arrive on the scene as quickly as possible.

Lie down with legs elevated. This position best maintains blood pressure and blood flow to the brain and vital organs.

Inject epinephrine. If the patient is a known anaphylactic, he or she is likely to have an epinephrine autoinjector medication close at hand. Known most commonly by the brand name EpiPen, this device can be used by any lay person by pressing the tip of the device to the outside of the thigh. It injects a dose of epinephrine, even through a layer of clothing. Some brands (like Auvi-Q) provide computerized voice instructions when opened. If the attack is occurring in a crowded room, such as a restaurant, someone else may be present who carries an epinephrine device. If the victim does not improve within five minutes after one shot, another dose can be given.

Continue providing emergency support until qualified personnel arrive. Inform them of the anaphylactic reaction so that they can administer epinephrine if this has not already been done.

Transport to an emergency room. Even if the patient receives an epinephrine injection and feels better, prompt transport to an emergency room is still critical. The epinephrine will wear off and the anaphylactic reaction may resume. Observation in an ER for eight hours or more is standard in case a relapse reaction occurs. It is common practice to administer steroids, antihistamines, and antacid medications for several days after an anaphylactic reaction to keep the allergic response suppressed.

Chronic, Recurrent Hives

If a specific physical cause is found, avoidance is the best measure. Chronic infections (if diagnosed by physical exam or testing) can be treated. For those without such a solution, medications should be considered. These can include antihistamines, leukotriene inhibitors (see page 69), steroids, and other advanced medications similar to those used in severe asthma (see page 63).

PREVENTING FUTURE ANAPHYLACTIC REACTIONS

Three factors are critical to preventing repeat episodes of severe anaphylaxis: identifying the cause, avoiding the cause, and keeping injectable epinephrine on hand.

Allergy Testing

In some cases, when the cause of the reaction is obvious, such as an insect sting or a meal of shellfish, you may believe that you don't need testing to confirm an obvious allergy. We agree in cases of mild, nonanaphylactic reactions. However, anyone who has suffered a severe reaction warrants testing, not only to confirm the suspected culprit, but to rule out other allergens as well. For example, if you reacted to almonds, you may want to test other tree nuts. If you are severely allergic to one food, you may want to rule out other common foods. And if you ate several suspected allergens, testing can narrow down the culprits. Your doctor will help you decide whether to do skin testing, blood testing, or both.

Avoiding Reexposure

Avoidance of allergic foods requires vigilance and preparedness, but it is manageable with the proper education. In general, you must learn how best to avoid dining scenarios that may lead to anaphylaxis, such as eating from a buffet or attending a potluck dinner. When dining out, inform your waiter of your allergies. Most restaurants now have allergen-specific menus. When you're shopping and eating at home, label reading is easier than ever; most labels clearly state which allergens are present in a food, right below the list of ingredients.

Insect allergies can also be prevented by following several basic precautions, discussed in Chapter 12. For example, learn which seasons and environments present the highest risk, and remove flowering plants around your yard to limit visiting bees.

If you have a medication allergy, such as to penicillin or latex, it's important to wear a medical alert bracelet at all times.

Injectable Epinephrine

Your doctor can prescribe an injectable epinephrine device, which will allow you to self-administer a shot of epinephrine in case of future anaphylactic reactions. An adult dose is indicated for anyone who weighs sixty-six pounds or more; a "junior" version with half the dose is available for infants and younger children. You should be prescribed two doses: one to keep with the patient at all times, and an extra to leave at a location where the patient spends much of his time, such as at school or work. Be sure to have your doctor or pharmacist demonstrate how to use it. Epinephrine is indicated only for true anaphylactic reactions. For mild reactions that involve only hives and do not progress to true anaphylaxis, epinephrine is not appropriate.

Consultation with an allergy specialist is important for anyone who has suffered an anaphylactic reaction, even if the culprit is obvious and you don't want testing; the specialist can fully consider all implications of the allergy and best advise you on testing and prevention.

Lowering Your Allergic Potential

The nutrition and lifestyle changes we present in Chapter 14 may have a positive impact on hives and lower your likelihood of a severe allergic reaction.

12

Insect Sting Allergies

Some reaction to insect stings is expected; most of us react to insect venom with swelling, redness, pain, or itching. Severe, anaphylactic reactions are uncommon, but when they do occur, they can be life-threatening and require prompt treatment (as detailed in the preceding chapter on anaphylaxis). This chapter describes what you and your family need to know if your allergic disorder involves stinging insects.

The primary type of insect that can trigger anaphylaxis comes from the group with the scientific name Hymenoptera. This group includes bees, wasps, yellow jackets, and hornets. Fire ants have also become an increasing problem in the southern part of the United States, particularly along the Gulf Coast.

IMMUNOLOGY OF INSECT STING REACTIONS

Insect stings cause reactions due to the venom that is injected into the skin during the sting. This venom contains enzymes and proteins that irritate the skin, as well as histamines that trigger a local allergic reaction. Most people experience this normal—and harmless—reaction to insect stings.

Those who are allergic, on the other hand, have IgE antibodies specific to the insect venom, and the allergic cascade begins as described in previous sections (see page 8). This reaction can remain limited to the part of the body near the sting, or it can travel through the bloodstream and trigger full anaphylaxis.

Biting insects (such as mosquitoes) don't inject venom from a stinger. Instead, they bite or puncture the skin with their mouths, and it is their saliva that triggers the swelling, redness, and itching. Anaphylactic reaction to biting insects is virtually unheard of.

SYMPTOMS OF INSECT STING ALLERGY

Everyone has at least a mild reaction to insect stings, involving itching, burning, redness, mild swelling, and pain, and this doesn't necessarily indicate an allergy. An allergy is suspected when a person has one of the following significant and bothersome reactions:

Swelling

An allergic person will experience swelling of the entire body part near the sting. For example, a sting on the hand will cause the entire hand to swell. Allergic swelling generally begins seven or eight hours after the sting, peaks between twenty-four and forty-eight hours after the sting, and then gradually subsides over the next week. This swelling can become quite tight, and it may involve an entire limb or large area surrounding a sting.

Redness

Swollen areas will generally look slightly redder than normal skin color; some will take on a darker red appearance. This redness is normal during the first forty-eight hours of an allergic response to a sting and generally does not indicate infection. As the swelling increases and the skin tightens, red areas may take on a whiter tone.

Anaphylactic Symptoms

As you learned in Chapter 11, a reaction that involves a second body system, other than just the skin, is categorized as an ana- phylactic reaction. Any respiratory, cardiovascular, or gastroin- testinal symptoms (see page 229) should be treated as an emergency. Fortunately, children have a much lower chance of insect anaphylaxis than do adults.

DO RED STREAKS INDICATE INFECTION?

Usually not. Red streaks that appear during the first forty-eight hours are generally part of the normal allergic reaction moving up your lymph ducts under the skin. Infection that is introduced through an insect sting or bite usually requires forty-eight hours or more to take hold and cause red streaks. Observe your child's affected area so you can accurately report on this to your doctor.

DIAGNOSING INSECT STING ALLERGY

If you or your child has had a nonanaphylactic but troublesome allergic reaction to an insect sting, a visit to your pediatrician or family doctor is warranted. If the reaction was anaphylactic (for which you probably received emergency care), an appointment with an allergy specialist is in order. Here is the general approach to diagnosing the allergy:

Nonanaphylactic Reactions

Those who have had a bothersome but nonanaphylactic allergic reaction to a first or second insect sting have a fairly low chance of ever suffering an anaphylactic reaction with future stings; some research demonstrates less than a 10 percent chance, and other research shows less than a 1 percent chance in children and a 3 percent chance in adults. Therefore, the general approach to such patients is to make sure they are aware of the allergy and to educate them on insect-avoidance precautions (see page 245). Epinephrine self-injections need not be prescribed, and no allergy testing is indicated.

One or More Anaphylactic Reactions

Those who have had an anaphylactic reaction should consult with an allergy specialist. IgE blood tests for specific insects can be done, as can skin tests, to document the exact type of insect allergy and help predict the likelihood of future anaphylactic reactions. Your doctor will discuss the relative value of each test. Epinephrine autoinjectors will likely be prescribed in case of future reactions, and the allergist can offer allergy shots (called venom immunotherapy) to reduce or eliminate the anaphylactic potential (see "Preventing Future Reactions," below).

TREATING INSECT STINGS

Treatment varies, depending on the severity of the reaction:

Nonanaphylactic Allergic Reactions

Swelling and redness can be minimized with cold compresses twenty minutes on/twenty minutes off for the first six hours, then less often as needed; a large Baggie with ice water works well. Over-the-counter oral antihistamines (see page 41) can also help. Hydrocortisone cream (also OTC) can reduce itching if needed. Be patient; improvement may be slow. Swelling may gradually worsen for a day or two before it begins to improve. As long as the discomfort is manageable, more aggressive therapy may not be needed. In cases of severe swelling that continues to worsen despite initial therapy, oral steroids can be prescribed for several days to halt the reaction.

Anaphylactic Reactions

Severe reactions should be treated according to the guidelines outlined on page 237.

PREVENTING FUTURE REACTIONS

While it is nearly impossible to completely avoid all stinging insects for the rest of your life, you can at least minimize the risk and be well prepared to treat a severe reaction. Allergy shots to decrease your reactivity to the venom can also be administered by a specialist.

Avoiding Bees and Their Friends

If you have an anaphylactic allergy, plan your outdoor time properly, and you'll be unlikely to get stung:

Proper clothing. Always wear shoes outside, as many stings come from stepping on a bee. Wear long sleeves and pants as often as the weather will allow, and avoid bright-colored clothing with floral patterns. Dull colors, like tan and green, or plain white, may be the least attractive to bees. Tight-fitting clothes are better, as insects may crawl inside loose-fitting clothes. Wear gloves when gardening or doing outdoor chores. Avoid perfumes, hair spray, and scented lotions.

Proper picnicking. Keep food put away in closed containers until it is time to eat. Do not use straws outdoors, as bees may hide inside. Drink from sealed containers instead of cans or open cups. Avoid soda and sweet juice when outside (water is healthier anyway).

Population control. Reduce the flowering plants and trees in your yard, or prune trees and plants before bee season (late summer and fall). I happen to have a large tree that attracts enormous numbers of bees in the late fall; we watch them swarm around all day long for about a month, and at least one finds its way into our house every day. If we remember to prune by the end of summer, we can avoid this buzzing nuisance. The only drawback is that bees are useful for cross-pollination of many other neighborhood trees, and reducing the naturally occurring bee population interferes with nature. But if you have a severe bee allergy, this is an important step. Hire a professional to remove any bee, wasp, or hornet nests from your yard.

Car safety. Keep windows rolled up, especially when parked.

Don't panic. If a bee lands on you or your child, avoid sudden movements and stay calm. Most insects will only sting in self-defense. Calmly remove the insect with a gentle but rapid swipe with a protected hand or object.

Don't Get Antsy

Most people are at least sensitive to fire ants; the large number of bites that occur when someone encounters fire ants can cause painful, blistery reactions. If you are allergic, however, these bites can result in anaphylaxis. Follow these precautions:

Proper care for fire ant bites. Each bite will usually blister, then fill with a thick, puslike fluid. Do not open the blisters. Wash with soap and water each day and keep the area clean. Allow the blisters to open and drain on their own. A scar is likely to remain afterward. Seek medical care if the bites, or the surrounding area, appear to become infected (symptoms of infection include spreading redness, heat, foul-smelling drainage, and fever).

Protective clothing. If you live in the South, especially around the Gulf Coast, be careful when working or playing outdoors. Fire ants live year-round, but they thrive during the spring, summer, and fall. Check the ground carefully before you settle into one spot, and look again a minute later to make sure you haven't stirred up a nest. Wear shoes and socks for protection, as well as gloves if you're working in the dirt.

Ant bait. If you find a nest in your yard, fire ant bait can be used, which will get carried into the nest and eliminate the queen ant.

Venom Immunotherapy

Similar to the allergy shots that are used to eliminate inhalant allergies, small doses of venom extract from bees, yellow jackets, hornets, wasps, or fire ants can be given weekly for about two months, then spaced out to monthly shots for a year or longer. These are only indicated for those with a history of severe allergic reactions and positive insect venom allergy tests. Research shows that some people will outgrow their insect allergy as they get older, and that this is far more likely if they receive venom immunotherapy. Your allergy specialist will discuss this with you further. See page 264 for more information.

In general, we encourage healthy lifestyle and dietary changes to help reduce a family's allergic disorders, as detailed in Chapter 14. However, insect venom allergy is a specific and unique problem, and little research exists on whether or not nutritional changes make a difference. We do not yet know how important the advice in Chapter 14 is for those with insect venom allergy.

13

Eliminating Inhalant Allergens: Dust, Mold, Pollen, Pets, and Allergy Shots

Those who are fortunate enough to discover their specific airborne allergens through testing can turn their energies to reducing or hopefully eliminating these annoyances from their lives forever. But it's not always an easy task. I am primarily allergic to dust mites. They will likely cause me some degree of trouble for the rest of my life because they are ubiquitous in our environment. But I can at least minimize exposure to the best of my ability so that I can be as symptom-free as possible. Our nutritional program has also, I believe, reduced my reactivity to dust.

Immunotherapy, otherwise known as allergy shots or oral desensitization therapy, can effectively eliminate a person's allergy to many of the inhalant allergens discussed in this chapter. If inhalant allergies are getting you down, see page 264 for details on when to consider this advanced treatment.

Reducing the inhalant allergens in your life takes time, money, and more time—but it's worth the effort. Although the initial nasal allergies caused by these inhalants may not seem serious, chronic nasal allergies can turn into asthma, and untreated asthma turns into decreased lung function decades later. Here are some guidelines to help you breathe more easily.

DUST MITES

Those who are allergic to dust aren't precisely allergic to the actual dust. Rather, they are allergic to the microscopic mites that live in the dust. These tiny organisms feed on the dead skin cells that slough off our bodies, so they tend to thrive wherever we spend a lot of time, such as in mattresses, pillows, couches, recliners, and carpets. And it's not just the mites themselves that people are allergic to—the allergenic mite proteins also exist in the mites' feces.

Dust mite allergy is diagnosed by blood or skin testing. The two species of dust mite that cause allergy are from the *Dermatophagoides* family; you will see them listed on your test form as *D. pteronyssinus* and *D. farinae*.

There are many ways you can minimize your exposure to dust mites, and some steps are more effective than others. You should focus your efforts and money on the most useful procedures first. Then pay more attention to the other steps as time goes by.

The Top Three Most Important Steps to Eliminating Dust

Here is what I have found to be the most valuable steps in reducing my exposure to dust mites and relieving my allergy symptoms:

Remove carpeting. Changing our entire house from wall-to-wall carpet to wood floors was expensive, but it made a tremendous difference for my asthma and allergies. We kept carpeting in one room, and sometimes when I walked into that room I could feel the change in the air; it felt thicker, and my nose started twitching right away. Symptoms would lessen for several days after vacuuming that room, but they always returned. Now that I've been gluten-free for a couple years, I don't notice these effects nearly as much. For those who test severely allergic to dust, I strongly recommend removing the carpeting as soon as you can.

Remodeling the entire house isn't always practical or affordable. If resources are limited, at least redo the bedroom of the allergy sufferer, and perhaps the family room or living room, where most of your time is spent. If carpeting is a must, use lower-pile commercial carpet, which traps less dust and fewer mites.

Aim for a dust-free bedroom. Focus on the mattress and bedding, as this is where we spend about one-third of our time. Encase mattresses, box springs, and pillows in mite-proof zippered covers. Wash blankets, sheets, and pillowcases in hot water (hotter than 130 degrees Fahrenheit) at least once a week to kill mites, and periodically vacuum the mattress. Keep closet doors closed to limit dust buildup in the closet. Be sure to damp-mop under and behind the bed weekly, as that's where dust loves to hide. Ensure that the rest of the bedroom is as dust-free as possible by removing the following objects, which harbor dust: cardboard boxes stacked in a corner or under the bed, bookshelves lined with books, heavy floor-length drapes and horizontal blinds, upholstered furniture, large house plants, fans, heavy wool blankets, and piles of stuffed animals. For children who need a few stuffed friends to keep them company at night, freeze the stuffed animals overnight once a week to kill the mites.

Down comforters and feather pillows may be a source of allergies as well, but not because of an allergy to the animal feathers themselves. Instead, these may harbor dust mites or mold spores. Allergy-proof covers should prevent symptoms.

Use an air purifier. I have tried various air purifiers over the years. I found that a HEPA filter unit (high-efficiency particulate air) helped somewhat. I tried several ionic purifiers but didn't find them effective. Then I was given a new ionic unit to try, and I found it a tremendous help in diminishing my dust allergy symptoms. It lasted several years, then had to be replaced, and I continue to use it every day. I don't know if this is the best air purifier out there, but it did happen to work well for my family and me. This sort of purifier can be found online from various companies, including EcoQuest (brand name Fresh Air) and Vollara (brand name FreshAir). See page 253 for more on air purifiers.

Other Useful Measures to Reduce Dust

As if the above steps aren't work enough, here are some other ways to reduce dust throughout the rest of the house:

Avoid upholstered furniture. Next to carpeting and mattresses, upholstered furniture is the greatest reservoir for dust mites. When we had our old couch, I could feel the dust surround me when I sat down. Vacuuming the couch and large reclining chairs helps, but it is difficult to keep up with this. What's better is to buy leather, vinyl, or other smooth-surfaced furniture that doesn't soak up the dust and mites in the first place.

Vacuum properly. Vacuum carpets and rugs about once a week. Vacuums throw a significant amount of dust and mites into the air, so be sure the dust-allergic member of the family isn't around for about a half hour from the time of vacuuming. If the allergy sufferer is the one doing the vacuuming, he should wear an appropriate mask to filter the air and use a vacuum equipped with a HEPA or other filtering mechanism to limit the amount of circulating dust.

Use vent filters. In addition to using an air purifier, place cheese-cloth or dust filters over air vents throughout the house. These will trap dust from the duct system before it is blown into the air when the heater or air conditioning is running. Change these filters, as well as the large ones in your central air system, every year or two to keep them fresh. Have your duct system profes-sionally cleaned every few years.

Monitor humidity. Dust mites and mold thrive on humidity. Use a humidity gauge and a dehumidifier as needed to keep indoor humidity between 25 and 40 percent.

HEPA VERSUS IONIC AIR PURIFIERS

There are several air-purifying technologies to choose from, and more may evolve in the coming years. The two primary types of air filters that most people use are HEPA filters and ionic filters; both types remove most allergens from the air, including dust, mold, pet dander, and pollen. HEPA (high-efficiency particulate air) filters are the most common. Small units will keep one room clean for a decent price; central units can be installed to filter the entire house, but these are fairly expensive. HEPA filters clean the dust and other particles out of the air by directly filtering the air as it passes through the unit. Ionic filters are a newer technology. They disperse ions (charged particles) in all directions from one small unit placed in a central location. One unit filters an average-sized house. These ions stick to most allergens in the air, causing them to fall to the ground so they won't be inhaled. Some filters attract the ion/allergen molecules back to the unit to be filtered. Some ionic filters also have an ozone feature, which cleans the air more thoroughly. Ozone, however, can irritate the lungs of asthmatics, so this feature should be turned off if anyone in the home has asthma.

Although air purifiers can be expensive, and many require periodic maintenance, if you find one that works well, it is worth the cost. Keep trying different brands and types until you find one that makes a difference.

MOLD

I also happen to have a mild mold allergy. During rainy weather, my nose begins to itch; then a sneezing, runny nose sets in for a few days as the moisture in the air and ground causes mold to blossom. My allergy was confirmed via testing many years ago. For me, mold isn't a big deal because my dust and pollen allergies override it. But for those who do have a primary mold allergy, the nasal and respiratory symptoms are very bothersome. Ongoing mold exposure can also contribute to chronic asthma and periodic asthma attacks.

The mold colonies release mold spores into the air, which are as light as dust. These spores float around, are inhaled, and then are deposited in the lining of the nose and lungs. For those with mold allergy, the spores trigger the classic IgE allergy response described on page 8, the same way dust and pollen trigger allergies. In addition, mold spores secrete chemicals that stimulate other immune cells to join in the reaction and program Th2 lymphocytes to remember the allergic sensitivity to that particular mold.

We are all exposed to mold every day. It is a normal part of our environment, both indoors and out, and for many of us it is harmless. Mold doesn't cause actual infections in healthy individuals. There are two primary ways in which mold does cause trouble: First, those who are allergic will experience allergy symptoms during particular times of the year or in certain locations. For people with severe mold allergy, symptoms can be just as troublesome as pet, pollen, or dust allergy and, in some cases, can be even worse. Second, household mold that grows over a long period because of slowly leaking water (such as a plumbing leak or a leaky roof), but remains undiscovered inside a wall, ceiling, floor, or cabinet, can release high levels of spores that will make everyone in the home experience sinus and respiratory symptoms, even if they are not typically allergic to mold.

It is useful to undergo allergy testing to determine whether mold is responsible for your symptoms. For people with chronic persistent allergies or asthma who initially test negative for mold allergy, periodic retesting is important to ensure that mold allergy is not contributing to your ongoing problems.

Species of Mold

There are numerous species of mold, and most people who are allergic are sensitive to only one or two species. You won't know which type you are allergic to unless you do allergy testing (skin or blood testing—see page 18). Just knowing that you are allergic to mold can allow you to take many general preventive measures (see below). Some molds tend to linger in certain areas of the house, thrive outdoors, or dwell in specific work environments. Determining which species is causing your allergies may help you track down where it is growing so that you can eliminate it. Here are the most common molds that cause allergic symptoms, and common locations where they can be found:

Alternaria. This mold grows on plants and thrives on decaying plant matter, particularly during the humid late-summer months and anytime moisture is abundant. On windy days, the spores blow around in high numbers; hot, dry climates allow the spores to easily disperse in the wind. Thunderstorms are known to kick up high levels of spores, which can trigger allergies and asthma attacks in those who are allergic. Spores will also blow indoors and cause symptoms.

Cladosporium. This shares many of the same properties as Alternaria mold, with the added ability to grow on indoor surfaces as well as outdoor.

Aspergillus. This thrives indoors where moisture collects, particularly in carpets, Sheetrock, and even dust. It loves hot, humid weather. Aspergillus causes a particularly severe respiratory illness, called allergic bronchopulmonary aspergillosis, in those with chronic lung disease (such as severe asthma or cystic fibrosis) or immune deficiency disorders; it does not occur in those with healthy lungs and immune systems.

Penicillium. This is an indoor mold, growing on spoiled food and numerous other types of organic material, including construction materials within walls and ceilings. It is the most common mold and grows on old bread, cheese, and fruit.

Mucor and **Rhizopus.** These grow in damp, indoor areas and thrive on old bread and sugary foods.

Stachybotrys. Known as black mold, this species feeds on damp building materials, so it thrives when indoor water leaks go unnoticed (as do many of the above molds). The spores are suspected of causing particularly severe respiratory symptoms and numerous other chronic symptoms; one extremely rare complication is bleeding within the lungs. Fortunately, most people who are exposed will suffer only mild allergy symptoms. Mold inspectors and professional mold removers tend to overemphasize the danger of black mold and scare clients unnecessarily. Yes, the mold is bothersome and should be removed, but no, it's not going to kill anybody in the meantime. Moving out of the home for a day or two while the worst of the mold is exposed and removed is usually appropriate.

There are numerous other species that may trigger allergies, and your doctor can provide you with any further details if necessary.

CHRONIC SINUS AND RESPIRATORY INFECTIONS: SUSPECT MOLD OVERLOAD

Although mold itself doesn't cause infection, high levels of continuous exposure to mold spores can trigger recurrent bacterial sinus and lung infections. Suspect mold when an entire family is ill for months on and off, especially during rainy seasons, after large water leaks, or when water damage is visible on walls or ceilings. Spores from the mold that is hidden within walls, cabinets, ceilings, or under the floor will leak into the air, and the daily exposure to this allergen will cause allergic symptoms at first, followed by bacterial illness in the entire family.

Reducing Exposure to Mold

For those who are mold-allergic, the following steps can reduce your exposure and symptoms:

Indoor mold

- Routinely clean mold-susceptible areas with a mold-killing disinfectant such as a 10 percent bleach solution. Areas include bathrooms, under sinks, shower curtains, window frames and sills, trash cans, refrigerator bottoms and rubber door gaskets, laundry rooms, basements, and even wallpaper.
- Maintain humidity between 25 and 40 percent within the home.
- Routinely clean cool-mist vaporizers and humidifiers.
- Mold-killing sprays can be sprayed into air-conditioning intake vents if you detect a musty odor.
- Use HEPA, ionic, or central air filters as discussed above in the dust reduction section, as these also eliminate mold spores.
- Night-lights in closets and bathrooms may reduce mold growth.
- Promptly repair or replace any water-damaged walls, floors, ceilings, carpets, or upholstered furniture. Wet ceiling tiles from roof leaks and damp Sheetrock are particularly prone to mold.

- Run the exhaust fan over the stove when boiling water and in the bathroom during hot showers to limit the humidity.
- Christmas trees tend to harbor mold. Clean out loose, damp pine needles before setting up your tree.

Outdoor mold

- Promptly remove damp piles of organic debris from the yard.
- Prune shrubbery and trees regularly to allow more mold-killing sunlight to shine around the outside of the house.
- Keep windows that are near large shrubs closed. Close up the house on windy days.
- Maintain adequate water drainage in the yard and around the house.
- Avoid visits to farms during harvest, and minimize time spent around hay, fruit trees, and freshly harvested grain.
- Avoid proximity to freshly cut grass and weeds, as these release mold spores into the air in addition to pollens. Compost heaps and mulch are havens for mold. Wear a filter mask over your mouth if such work is necessary.
- Stay clear of damp piles of leaves. Even hiking in woods surrounded by decaying fall leaves is likely to trigger symptoms in those who are allergic.
- Mold thrives on moist outdoor wood furniture. Keep such furniture covered to prevent moisture buildup, and periodically clean it with a bleach solution.

Professional Mold Removal

Professional mold inspectors can be hired to test for, and eradicate, mold. This is money well spent when your situation warrants it. Large areas of mold contamination from water damage are the most common scenario that requires professional help, especially when the mold has been hidden behind walls for a while. Those with chronic asthma who require ongoing aggressive medical therapy should have their home inspected to be sure mold isn't a contributing factor. Those who test highly allergic to mold should follow all of the above precautions, particularly those that apply to your specific mold; if symptoms persist, a professional inspection may be useful.

DON'T FORGET COCKROACH ALLERGY

Although we don't like to think about it, cockroaches are unwanted but inevitable houseguests in some parts of the country. Their saliva, feces, and shed skins are allergens for a small proportion of the population. Roaches also frequent warehouses and storage facilities and may trigger allergies in those who work in such places. Children who experience allergies only at school may be reacting to these insect residents. Roach allergy is diagnosed with routine allergy testing. If you live or work around roaches and test allergic, take the following steps to minimize your exposure:

- Keep eating areas clean, store food in closed containers, wash dishes promptly, and empty the trash routinely.
- Place bait traps in appropriate areas.
- Hire a professional exterminator to routinely treat as needed.
- Do not store cardboard boxes, newspapers, and paper bags in the home.
- Ensure that cracks, crevices, and plumbing fixtures are properly sealed.

POLLEN

Ah, the great outdoors! A stroll through the woods, a long backyard nap in a lounge chair, or a picnic in the park are all enjoyable pastimes...unless you have pollen allergy. And blustery days are the worst for this allergy. I have some pollen allergy that used to bother me considerably during certain seasons, and I relied heavily on allergy meds. With all of the nutritional and allergy-prevention changes I've made in recent years, I no longer suffer during any particular pollen seasons.

On page 32 you read about when to suspect pollen as a cause of nasal allergies; pollen also contributes to chronic asthma, as well as acute asthma attacks. Pollen allergy is usually diagnosed with skin or blood testing, which tests for a wide range of plant pollens.

An interesting phenomenon, called oral allergy syndrome, occurs in some people with pollen allergy. This is a cross-reaction between pollen and food allergies. See page 194 for details on which foods might cause such reactions.

Types of Pollen

Pollen is made up of tiny particles that are shed from plants as part of their reproductive process. Plants release most of their pollen in the morning, but wind disperses it throughout the day. There are three primary types of pollen:

Tree pollen. Most fruit trees and some pine trees do not produce pollens that are allergenic. Most other trees, however, do, including junipers, cedars, elms, birches, maples, some pines, and many others. Each type of tree has a relatively short period each year during which it releases its pollen; many do so in the late winter into spring. The time spent with allergy symptoms may be short for those with only one allergy. Some trees pollinate at other times throughout the year, though, so those with multiple allergies may suffer during more than one season.

Grass pollen. Grasses release their pollen during growing seasons. In the South and on the southwest coast of the United

States, Bermuda grass is predominant, and it releases pollen throughout the year because it grows continuously. The northern half of the United States has a variety of grasses, including timothy and bluegrass; these grow primarily during the spring and summer and therefore predictably cause allergies during these seasons. High-elevation areas of the country have very little grass pollen in the air.

Weed pollen. Most weed pollens don't cause allergies. Of the ones that do, ragweed is the most common and most bothersome cause of seasonal nasal allergies. Ragweed grows abundantly in the midwestern plains and eastern agricultural states where soil is routinely cultivated, and it releases pollen during the late summer and early fall. Ragweed's association with seasonal nasal allergies around farming communities has prompted the lay term *hay fever.* A variety of other weeds affect other regions of the United States.

Testing to determine specific pollen allergies is useful in two ways: First, it may provide specific information that allows you to limit your exposure and predict seasonal variations. Second, it helps determine whether or not you would benefit from allergy shots (see page 264).

Reducing Exposure to Pollen

Those who are allergic don't have to be left to the mercy of the wind, weather, and season. Here are the steps you can take to minimize your exposure to pollen:

Monitor pollen counts. Some pollens are seasonal; others are year-round. If you test allergic to one or more, your doctor will tell you what seasons will trouble you the most. You can also monitor pollen counts on various websites and news stations, and with apps on your mobile device. When you know you are in for a bad day, week, or month, step up your sinus health measures, discussed on page 40, to minimize the pollen's effects, and take allergy medication as needed. Take extra care with the rest of our suggested steps in this section when pollen counts are high.

Use air purifiers. Ionic or HEPA air cleaners and central filters, discussed on page 253, clean many of the pollen particles out of the air. You will likely keep one running year-round if you are allergic to dust; if pollen is your only problem, you will prolong your purifier's life by only running it on days with high pollen counts and during your troublesome seasons.

Close windows. Close the windows when pollen is high. Keep car windows rolled up when driving around town. Use air conditioning as needed, and make sure any outside air is properly filtered as it passes through your central air system.

Decontaminate. At the end of each day, remove pollen from your body by taking a shower, washing your hair, and putting on a clean set of clothes or pajamas. Put used clothing directly into the laundry room. Hang jackets and hats in a mudroom or hallway closet, and periodically wash jackets during allergy season. Do not bring any outdoor clothing into the bedroom.

Play indoors. If you or your child has a predictable seasonal allergy to a certain tree, type of grass, or specific weed that you can identify around your house or in your neighborhood, learn what time of year it pollinates and limit outdoor play during such times (if the severity of symptoms warrants such a precaution). If allergic to grass, stay clear of freshly mowed lawns.

PET ALLERGY

Those who are allergic to pets and other animals are allergic to the dried flakes of skin that shed from the animals, called *dander;* it is not the actual pet hair itself that triggers the allergy. Animal saliva and urine can also contain allergens. Dander particles are extremely small and light, so they remain suspended in household air for long periods. All dogs and cats shed skin cells, so even short-haired breeds, and so-called hypoallergenic breeds, can trigger allergies. New research has prompted many allergists to agree that there is no longer any such thing as a hypoallergenic breed of dog.

It isn't clearly understood why some people are born with, or later develop, pet allergy. Genetics likely plays a major role, and environmental factors contribute as well. Growing up with pets seems to help reduce allergic disorders in general; but pet allergy seems to occur independently of whether or not the person grows up around animals.

Pet allergy is diagnosed with skin or blood testing. If the allergy is confirmed, the best long-term solution is to find that pet a new home and welcome other types of pets into your life. Still, we understand that family pets are so deeply loved by adults and children alike that some will choose to keep a beloved pet. The severity of allergy symptoms must be considered in such cases; if severe asthma is the result of a pet allergy, retaining the pet is probably not the best choice. Pet-allergic families who don't have animals should periodically expose new infants and young children to dogs and cats to induce immune tolerance and to help them benefit from the allergy-prevention effects of animal exposure. Here are some ways you can minimize exposure to the dander:

- Routinely clean house to remove accumulated pet dander.
- Use a properly filtered vacuum (HEPA or other) to reduce the dispersal of pet dander.

- Keep the allergic person's bedroom door closed so the pet doesn't shed in the bedroom.
- Keep windows open and the home well ventilated (assuming outdoor allergens are not a problem).
- Use air purifiers (see page 253) to remove dander from the air.
- Routinely wash the pet to minimize shedding. Perform all brushing and grooming outdoors.
- Keep pets off upholstered furniture, where shed skin can accumulate.
- Minimize the amount of carpeting and rugs in the home, as these accumulate dander.
- Use antihistamine medications, a safe and effective treatment, when pet exposure is necessary.
- Try natural, homeopathic oral sprays available for pet allergies; these may be effective for some people.

If all else fails, allergy shots can effectively reduce dog and cat allergies. See below.

IMMUNOTHERAPY: ALLERGY SHOTS, SUBLINGUAL IMMUNOTHERAPY, AND ORAL DESENSITIZATION

Immunotherapy is an approach that lowers the immune system's allergic responsiveness to allergens. Classically, allergy shots have been the primary method used in the United States. Oral desensitization (feeding tiny amounts of an allergic food in gradually increasing amounts) for peanuts is a growing practice, and milk and egg desensitization research looks promising (but is not yet approved). Sublingual immunotherapy (dissolving allergen tablets under the tongue) has been a standard alternative to shots for many years in other countries. It has just been FDA approved for some grass allergens (see below), and more applications should follow in the years to come.

Allergy Shots

The thought of taking allergy shots week after week, month after month, for years and years is daunting to most people. This bad rap prevents many from considering this step, but we encourage patients to consult with an allergist to consider this therapy under the right circumstances.

Allergy shots are available for the following inhalant allergens:

- Grass pollen
- Ragweed pollen (and some other weeds)
- Some tree pollen
- Cat dander
- Dog dander
- Dust mites
- Cockroaches
- Molds (Alternaria, Aspergillus, and Penicillium)

Allergy shots are also available for insect venom stings (by bees, yellow jackets, hornets, wasps, or fire ants).

The Immunology of Immunotherapy

Immunotherapy administers ever-increasing amounts of allergens to the body. This causes an initial rise in IgE antibody levels to that allergen (as expected), but often without triggering any noticeable allergic reactions because the amount of allergen is so minimal. Rarely, a person will have an allergic reaction to the shot, and the allergy specialist will be on hand to treat any emergency situations. The body eventually becomes less sensitive to that allergen, and IgE levels diminish over time and end up at a level much lower than baseline. In addition, the immune system also responds by producing IgG antibodies to the allergen, which may indicate tolerance. Furthermore, the Th2 lymphocytes, which are responsible for programming allergic responses, decrease. This immunological process is very complex and is not yet completely understood. The end result for many is elimination of the allergy.

Who Should Try Immunotherapy

As previously stated, research has shown that those who undergo immunotherapy for chronic nasal allergies not only find relief from their nasal symptoms, but also have a significantly lower rate of later developing asthma *if* they begin immunotherapy before seeing any signs of asthma. In addition, those with only one primary allergy who receive allergy shots are less likely to become allergic to other major allergens later. This is true for both children and adults, and some allergists will consider immunotherapy in children as young as three years of age. Even those who have already developed asthma can benefit from allergy shots, if their primary allergens are on the above list.

Allergy Shot Ingredients

It is only natural for parents to wonder what is in allergy shots. After all, if you are going to allow these injections to be given to your child, or yourself, week after week, month after month, you want to know that there are no harmful ingredients. There are five major manufacturers of allergy shots in the United States. We have reviewed the product inserts of many of their shots, and we've found that they are almost identical. These shots do not contain any harmful chemicals or unusual ingredients, and they contain no mercury (thimerosal). We believe they are safe for human use.

Allergy shots are made up of two primary ingredients: the allergen itself (pollen, animal dander, etc.) and glycerin, along with some electrolytes and saline solution. Some contain traces of acetone. None of these ingredients are harmful or dangerous. If concerned, you can ask your allergist to review the ingredients in the specific product he or she uses.

We recommend patients consider allergy shots if ongoing allergies don't adequately resolve with prevention and treatment steps.

Sublingual Immunotherapy

This therapy for inhalant allergies is an emerging practice in Europe and other countries, but it is not yet widely accepted in the United States. Newly approved sublingual allergens for grass and ragweed are now available through your allergist. Researchers are still studying sublingual therapy for dust mites, other pollens, peanuts, milk, cats, and other allergens. Periodically ask your allergy specialist if such therapies are yet available.

14

Our Prescription for Optimum Immune Health: Healing and Preventing Allergic Disorders

In your journey through this book, you have learned that allergic disorders come in all shapes and sizes. From eczema and hives to a runny nose and cough, from gastrointestinal problems and behavioral challenges to wheezing attacks and life-threatening anaphylaxis, allergies take a profound toll on our health and well-being. Treatments are unique to each particular allergic problem: eczema has topical therapy, nasal allergy has nasal sprays and pills, asthma has inhalers, and food allergy has life-saving adrenaline shots.

But all allergic disorders have one thing in common: the immune system is out of balance. The allergic branch of the immune system is revved up and out of control in all of these disorders, and it needs to be brought back into balance so that symptoms abate, quality of life improves, and long-term health complications disappear. Achieving immune balance should be a primary goal for every person with allergies, from the youngest infant to the oldest adult. This chapter describes how you can bring your immune system into better balance, no matter what allergic disorder ails you.

You might be wondering about subsequent children who have yet to join your growing family. Can you lower their risk of carrying on the family tradition of allergies? Yes, you can. Our prescription includes preventive steps that can help avert allergic disorders before they begin.

Our healing "prescription" has been formulated from decades of experience in the Sears family pediatrics office. It's a science-based prescription that is guaranteed to lessen the severity of allergies. Every family can follow it, and it will shape your family's health habits for life.

But our prescription involves significant effort on your part. It takes our Pills and Skills approach to therapy to the highest level. Every family *can* do it, but it's not an easy pill to swallow. We ask you to put all your skills to work for yourself, your child, and your family. The allergy "pills" you've read about throughout this book bring relief, but they don't bring *resolution*. If you stay committed to our prescription for optimum immune health, you will see results, and your family's health will reap the benefits.

Our prescription has many components. Some are simple lifestyle and environmental changes to clean up your life. Reducing stress and finding a positive attitude (using mind over your wheezing and itchy body) are a key element. Exercise must be a regular routine to mobilize your body's natural immune-balancing hormones. Making wise health care choices during pregnancy, infancy, and childhood will also influence allergic risk. But the most significant factor, the one that has the most profound effect on the immune system, is nutrition and gut health. Protecting the intestinal health of infants and young children is critical, and eating more immune-balancing foods and fewer inflammatory foods in the early years and through adulthood is the wisest form of preventive medicine.

The gut is the largest immune organ in the body; there are more immune cells in the gut than in the rest of the body combined. So this is where our efforts to achieve immune balance must begin. Once gut health is restored, the immune balance in the rest of the body will soon follow. We will spend most of this chapter sharing several cutting-edge ideas regarding nutrition and allergies that will help you achieve resolution of your allergic disorders.

For some families with milder allergic disorders, our advice can be summed up in one sentence, probably similar to what your mom "prescribed" years ago: "Eat more fruits and vegetables and go outside and play!" We wish it were that simple for everybody. Families who are challenged by moderate and severe allergic problems will have to dig deeper into this chapter to discover the more extensive healing solutions.

In addition to nutrition and lifestyle changes, there is a world of natural treatments for allergic disorders that are worth exploring. Many herbal remedies and some alternative medical practices have good research to support them, but some do not. At the end of this chapter, we present numerous alternative options — ones that we believe have merit — for you to consider.

HEALING AND PREVENTING ALLERGIC DISORDERS DURING PREGNANCY AND INFANCY

The two most common allergic challenges during infancy are eczema and intestinal problems. These are often caused by food allergies, and you have already worked through those sections of this book. Respiratory disorders may begin during infancy as well, although these are more of a challenge during later childhood. This section provides several additional steps you can take to ensure your infant's immune health. If you are still struggling to find answers, these additional steps may uncover the missing key for you and your baby. If you've already found resolution to your baby's allergies, this information will help you maintain your child's health. These steps will also be critical for you to follow with subsequent babies to help prevent a repeat of your family's allergic disorders.

The single most important factor during infancy is to preserve the integrity of the intestines and intestinal immune system. To achieve this, an infant's introduction to life must be as natural as possible. A baby's gut and immune system must be allowed to mature with minimal insults. Here are the most important preventive steps you can take with your new baby.

Natural Childbirth

The first step in achieving optimal intestinal immune balance is to have a healthy vaginal delivery with appropriate medical guidance. You've already learned that our healthy intestinal bacteria play a crucial role in our immune health, and an imbalance in these bacteria sets the stage for allergic disorders. Vaginal delivery provides a baby with his very first "immunization" — a dose of his mom's healthy bacteria (known as probiotics), which live in the birth canal. At first glance, this seems counterintuitive. Why would such bacteria be good for a baby? But nature designed it so that these healthy bacteria initially come from the mother. Research shows that the healthy bacteria that live in an infant's gut match the bacteria that live in a mom's birth canal. These bacteria go on to multiply and colonize the entire intestinal system and set the stage for a lifetime of intestinal health.

Some infants, out of medical necessity, must be delivered by cesarean section. This medical procedure provides lifesaving care for distressed infants and moms every day and prevents very serious birth complications. However, it deprives the infant of Mom's healthy vaginal bacteria. Instead, the bacteria from Mom's skin and from the hospital environment make up the initial species that colonize the rest of baby's gut. Research has confirmed that babies born by C-section go on to have a less diverse population of healthy bacteria in the gut during infancy and have a higher chance of eczema and asthma. Fortunately, breast milk provides some healthy probiotics regardless of birth method. While most infants born by C-section will go on to live healthy lives without allergic disorders, this lack of healthy intestinal bacteria does raise the risks compared to infants born vaginally. (For the latest research on ways to increase a mother's chances of delivering vaginally, read: *The Healthy Pregnancy Book* by Sears and Sears, Little, Brown, 2013.)

Some medical practitioners advise the introduction of supplemental probiotics for infants if born by C-section. Research has demonstrated benefits in reducing colic and allergic disorders, but this research isn't conclusive. While not as healthy as Mom's natural probiotics from the birth canal, supplemental probiotics may be useful. See page 300 for more information on choosing an infant probiotic. Researchers have also begun to look at administering doses of Mom's vaginal flora to baby using cotton swabs after a C-section to try to simulate a natural birth exposure. While not yet approved, this commonsense approach may end up providing babies with a good dose of allergy prevention. Even the flora in saliva may help; research shows that placing a pacifier into a parent's mouth prior to giving it to baby reduces asthma and eczema. The same should be true when baby sucks on a parent's finger.

The Issue of Antibiotics During Labor

Intravenous antibiotics are routinely given during many vaginal deliveries to prevent a newborn infection called Group B strep, or GBS. This species of *Streptococcus* bacteria lives in the birth canal of 25 to 40 percent of women (research varies). After Mom's water breaks, these bacteria can move up into the uterus, multiply, and cause a very serious, even life-threatening, infection in Mom or baby. This is primarily a risk when labor lasts for twelve or more hours after Mom's water breaks, as shorter labors rarely allow enough time for the bacteria to move up to the uterus and cause infection. Because of the potential severity of GBS infections, IV antibiotics are advised during labor for all women who test positive with a vaginal swab—a practice that saves countless lives every year.

But there's a drawback to this practice as well. These IV antibiotics reduce the levels of healthy bacteria in the birth canal, meaning the baby doesn't get an optimal exposure to healthy bacteria during vaginal delivery. The antibiotics flow through the placenta into the baby and disrupt the growth of the healthy bacteria that try to colonize baby's gut after birth. They can also cause yeast overgrowth in Mom's breasts and in baby's mouth and gut, which further interferes with healthy bacterial colonization.

(With C-sections, moms are given an IV dose after the baby is delivered to help prevent postoperative wound infection. These antibiotics don't enter the baby directly, so there is less initial disruption of the baby's system. But the ensuing yeast infection in Mom's breasts can be bothersome to both Mom and baby.)

The vaginal-birth antibiotics are necessary for women who test positive for GBS because GBS infections can be so devastating. But the reality is that most infants who are born less than twelve hours after Mom's water breaks will not be affected by Mom's GBS bacteria. Is it worth it to disrupt the healthy bacterial colonization process in these babies and increase the long-term risk of allergic disorders, or is there a better way to determine which GBS-positive moms really need these antibiotics? Perhaps a logical compromise would be to not give antibiotics to moms whose water stays intact throughout labor, thus allowing the healthy establishment of gut bacteria in more babies. But the danger of GBS must be weighed in this decision. Parents should discuss this dilemma with their health care provider and make an informed decision.

When such antibiotics are necessary, we advise Mom and baby to use probiotic supplementation to help counteract the effects on the gut. See page 300 for details.

Breastfeed Exclusively

Medical research is very clear that exclusive breastfeeding lowers the risk of allergies. Colostrum (the first few days of breast milk) has numerous healthy components that prepare baby's intestines for digestion and establish a healthy and balanced immune system. Breast milk is uniquely suited to be easily digested, it contains healthy probiotic bacteria that perform crucial immune functions in the gut, and it has growth factors that feed a baby's own healthy probiotic bacteria. Also, it's loaded with IgA antibodies and several other types of immune cells to protect a baby from infection. It's human milk for human babies, and it is the healthiest option for infants.

Exclusive breastfeeding means just that. *Exclusive.* Research shows that just one bottle of formula disrupts the integrity of the intestines for weeks. The most likely time when an infant will be offered formula is during the first few days of life, while waiting for Mom's milk to come in; many hospitals push formula on vulnerable new mothers at that time. The American Academy of Pediatrics advises against giving a baby any formula in the early days if breastfeeding is planned, unless there is a definite medical need. Babies are designed to begin the first few days of life on colostrum only; they need very little milk and will thrive as soon as Mom's milk comes in on day three or four after birth.

Moving forward through baby's first year, it's tempting to supplement breast milk with formula to give Mom a break. Many formulas now have probiotics, but don't be fooled: these probiotics are not nearly as useful as the natural ones in Mom's milk. Unless there is a definite need for supplementation, formula is not advised, especially if allergies already run in the family.

Prolonged breastfeeding for two years or more, along with the proper introduction of foods after six months, is the best nutritional prevention for allergies. Furthermore, research shows that infants who are still breastfeeding when eventually first exposed to gluten have a 50 percent lower risk of eventually developing celiac disease.

Treating Breast Infections

Some moms will experience a breast infection called mastitis. This occurs when a milk duct within the breast becomes plugged and bacteria grow within the stagnant milk, causing a painful, hard, hot lump within the breast and a fever with flulike symptoms. The standard medical approach to these infections is to simply give Mom a course of antibiotics. No harm done, right? Well, you've already learned how disruptive antibiotics can be to a baby's developing gut bacteria. When Mom takes a weeklong course of oral antibiotics, the baby is exposed to small doses through the breast milk for the week as well. This kills some of baby's healthy germs and can trigger yeast overgrowth.

Most cases of early mastitis can be successfully treated without antibiotics by instead using hot compresses and gentle massage to drain the plugged ducts. Consultation with a lactation specialist can help a mom through this process and can prevent future plugged ducts. Antibiotics should be reserved for severe cases with persistent fever that don't respond to nonmedical therapy, and they should be taken along with probiotic therapy.

Avoiding Antibiotic Overuse in Infancy and Toddlerhood

New medical guidelines prompt doctors to use antibiotics more cautiously, especially in infants. However, many patients still pressure their health care providers for unnecessary prescriptions. Antibiotics are important when needed, but as you've already learned, they have one major drawback that can exacerbate allergic disorders: antibiotics kill many of the healthy bacteria that live in our gut. And when the healthy germs are killed, yeast and antibiotic-resistant bacteria build up and secrete numerous toxins that irritate our GI system. The immune system reacts throughout the body to these unhealthy germs and toxins, and the allergic branch flares up and creates even more inflammation. Research on antibiotics during infancy has revealed two important factors: (1) the earlier a first antibiotic is given, the greater the risk of future allergic disorders, and (2) several courses of antibiotics create a higher risk than just one or two. New research shows that multiple antibiotic courses prior to age two almost doubles the risk of asthma.

We are certainly not opposed to proper use of antibiotics. We used to prescribe them almost every day in our office; we do so less often now. A single course of antibiotics is generally well tolerated in an older infant who has already established a healthy immune balance in the gut, and supplemental probiotics can help minimize the effects.

What we advise against is the repeated use of unnecessary antibiotics. If the above-mentioned inflammatory process is repeated over and over again, allergic disorders will soon follow. In our practice, we use antibiotics only when necessary, and we use science-based natural treatments whenever possible. Two of our favorites, which are supported by some preliminary research (although not conclusive enough to become mainstream), are mullein–garlic oil eardrops to relieve ear pain during ear infections, and natural herbal remedies for colds, coughs, and sinus infections. We also use immune-boosting supplements for those with recurrent infections. And we are very selective in prescribing antibiotics during infancy when the gut and immune system are being established. Visit AskDrSears.com and DrBobsDaily .com for more information on natural treatments and ways to boost the immune system.

Probiotic Supplementation for Mom and Baby

While some research does not demonstrate any benefit, other studies show that supplementing a mom with probiotics throughout pregnancy and giving a baby daily probiotics help reduce allergic disorders, particularly eczema. We now recommend this preventive therapy to the allergic families in our practice. See page 300 for details on choosing a probiotic.

THE SEARS PARENTING LIBRARY

For more information on making wise and healthy decisions regarding childbirth, see *The Healthy Pregnancy Book* in the Sears Parenting Library.

Need help and support with achieving long-term breastfeeding success? Check out *The Breastfeeding Book.*

The Portable Pediatrician book in the Sears Parenting Library provides detailed guidelines on treating infections appropriately, minimizing antibiotics, and boosting the immune system.

Solve Breast Milk or Formula Intolerance Quickly

Some infants are sensitive to certain food proteins in Mom's milk. And infants who are formula-fed are often sensitive to cow's milk or other formula ingredients. These situations can cause eczema, colic, and intestinal problems. Chapter 7 provides a detailed approach to solving these issues. We offer a brief reminder here to work through these issues quickly so that you can better establish a healthy gut during early infancy.

Proper Introduction of Baby Food

In Chapter 6 we provide a unique and updated look at how to safely introduce foods to a growing baby in a way that best reduces the risk of allergies. Review this information as you begin solid foods with your subsequent babies.

Integrative Medicine

An emerging type of medical practice that more and more physicians are turning to is called integrative medicine. It's a combination of mainstream and natural medical approaches to health care. Such physicians limit antibiotic use and incorporate science-based natural treatments into their practice, and they pay special attention to intestinal health during infancy and childhood. If your family is challenged with allergic disorders, seek out an integrative medical practitioner in your area so you can make the best choices possible for your family.

LIFESTYLE CHANGES TO HEAL AND PREVENT ALLERGIC DISORDERS IN CHILDREN AND ADULTS

Beyond infancy, numerous factors can influence the risk of allergic disorders. Limiting antibiotics continues to be a priority, though it isn't as critical as it is in the first two years. You have likely already diagnosed food allergies and other allergic triggers at this stage. You are now at the point where either you have tried everything and your problems have not been adequately resolved, or you are looking to take preventive steps in your family to help reduce overall allergic risks. A myriad of healthy lifestyle and nutritional choices can help ensure your family's long-term health.

Slow Down

The first step in achieving immune balance is to examine your own lifestyle. Are you too busy? Do you have a high-stress job? Do you spend most of your time indoors? Do you run around all day caring for others without taking care of yourself? Are you overly committed to activities and organizations outside the home that take up much of your time and energy?

After taking a look at your own lifestyle, you should examine the lifestyles of your children with allergies. Do they sit inside all day watching TV and playing video games? Are they too stressed about school? Are they getting sick too often and overloaded with antibiotics? Do you spend enough time together as a family, relaxing, playing games, and having fun?

For any chronic illness, it pays to take a step back and examine your lifestyle. Let's consider the typical middle-aged American male who's just had his first heart attack. His high-stress job, poor diet, and lack of exercise combined to close off his coronary arteries and trigger the heart attack. After surgery and recovery, can this man go back to his old lifestyle? Not if he wants to live. He must reduce stress, eat properly, and begin an exercise program if he wants to live a long and happy life.

The same is true for allergic disorders. You must do more than just avoid the allergens and take a daily pill. Sometimes we just have to slow down, take a deep breath, and evaluate what's important to us. And nothing is more important than family. You may have to work hard, and you will have some stress, but the steps we advise in this section will help you find the right balance for immune and allergic health.

Go Outside

Remember when you were a child and you roamed free around the neighborhood with your friends, just barely making it home in time for dinner? We do. Spending time outside is good for the mind and the body, and it's good for the immune system. Here is how:

Immune tolerance. Picture this scenario: An infant is born and spends his first three years of life playing mostly indoors, where life is clean and safe. Then he enters preschool, where he is suddenly exposed to germs, pollens, plants, pets, and dozens of other allergens his immune system has never seen before. He is more likely to react to these allergens because they are foreign to his immune system.

Instead, consider the infant who is exposed to many allergens early in life while the immune system is developing. Mom takes baby to the park almost every day. They visit petting zoos and the local organic farm. They breathe in some pollens and natural molds. They play in grass and dirt and crawl through the bushes. Baby's immune system learns that these allergens are a normal part of life and becomes tolerant of them.

Vitamin D. This hormone is activated in the skin by natural sunlight, and it then flows throughout the body to help balance the immune system and prevent numerous chronic conditions. Several research studies show that vitamin D deficiency is a risk factor for allergic disorders. To maintain healthy vitamin D levels in the body, children and adults should spend a few hours each day outside, without sunscreen (which prevents vitamin D activation). Avoid sunburn by limiting sun exposure in the middle hours of the day.

If spending this much time outdoors isn't practical for your lifestyle or climate, supplement with vitamin D drops or tablets. See page 299 for details on dosing.

Enjoying real nature. The medical community has recently established a new condition called nature deficit disorder. Children and adults who don't spend enough time outdoors have more stress, more behavioral problems, and more mood and learning disorders. These stresses also contribute to immune imbalance. In addition to spending more time in the backyard and playing around the neighborhood, plan routine nature walks and more adventurous outings in forests, on hills and mountains, and in other locales that help you and the family "get away from it all."

For an insightful read about how scenes of nature mellow a quirky immune system, check out *Your Brain on Nature,* by Harvard neuroscientist Dr. Eva Selhub and Alan C. Logan.

Consider a Major Move

Living in a big city can take its toll on lung health. In 1981, our family moved to smoggy Los Angeles, and we soon realized our mistake. We remember having to stop Little League games because the air made the young players wheeze. My asthma eased once we moved to the clean seaside air of San Clemente, California. Sometimes families with asthma have to move to achieve healthier lives.

Perhaps your family's allergies are specific to where you live, caused by regional pollens or mold. If your symptoms are severe and chronic enough, it may be time to move to a new town, or even a new state if it's feasible. Consult with your allergist to determine whether your allergies may be significantly lessened in certain parts of the country.

If you do relocate, make sure your new neighborhood is far away from major highways, freeways, and factories. The air pollution in such areas can have a significant impact on sinus and lung health.

A Healthy Home Environment

If nasal allergies and asthma are your family's primary challenges, routinely read through Chapter 13, "Eliminating Inhalant

Allergens: Dust, Mold, Pollen, Pets, and Allergy Shots," for a reminder on how to minimize dust, mold, and other irritants. It pays to keep your home clean and allergen-free.

Also remember that smoking and allergic disorders don't mix. If someone in the home has allergies, smoking cessation is an absolute must. Secondhand cigarette smoke is a direct cause of asthma in children, and it also contributes to the many other allergic disorders.

Techniques to Lower Stress

Stress increases immune system dysfunction, wheezing, and inflammation. You start to wheeze and feel like you're not getting enough air; then you start worrying about the wheezing and further constrict your airways. A new field of scientific research called psychoneuroimmunology—that's a mouthful—is revealing that when we turn down stress, we improve our immune system balance. Happy thoughts trigger happy neurohormones, which reduce neuroinflammation and help balance the immune system. The sooner you and your child master "mind over allergies," the faster those allergies will lessen. Here are some stress-busting tools for you to consider:

Tame the trigger. While stress-triggering allergic reactions are more common in adults, they do happen to kids as well. What worry might set off the wheeze, itch, or drip? Is it school exams or a family fight? Once you've identified the stressor, remove the trigger as best you can.

Teach mood switching. When you or your child feels a wheeze coming on, fill your minds with happy thoughts. Call them "instant replays": recall hitting a home run, dancing onstage, or playing soccer. Teach your child to fill her mind with her favorite memories and replay them as soon as she feels an allergic reaction starting. One of our patients with severe asthma would replay his favorite family beach scene memories as soon as he felt a wheeze coming on, which would distract him from worrying about his wheeze. Read a story, give a massage, turn on some music, start quietly singing, or do something else that lifts the family mood.

Trash negative thoughts. Another child-appropriate way to explain mood switching is to focus on getting rid of the *ants* (*a*utomatic *n*egative *t*houghts) in your brain. Encourage kids to quickly throw the "ants" outside. Teach your young kids to "throw the thought into the trash and watch the trash truck take it away." Tell your older child: "As soon as a disturbing thought enters your mind, quickly 'trash' it like you would send junk e-mails into the trash bin on your computer."

We frame it for our children this way: "Negative thoughts are like footprints on the sand. Allow the surf of happy thoughts to wash them away immediately. If you don't, the sand may turn to concrete. These negative thoughts could last forever and become part of your brain."

Humor heals. Yes, laughter is the best medicine, especially when allergies strike. Laughter raises the blood level of natural germ-fighting and immune-balancing cells, and it speeds healing. That's why smart Dr. Mom smiles as she places the nebulizer in the mouth of her wheezing child.

Music heals. Call it "iPod therapy" or "Try your iPod for your wheezing bod." Music helps the body release happy and healing anti-inflammatory hormones.

In through the nose. New research reveals that nasal breathing stimulates the lining of the nasal passages to release a natural antiallergy biochemical called nitric oxide, which acts like an anti-inflammatory for the nose and a vasodilator for the lungs, helping the blood vessels in the lungs carry more oxygen. Try this exercise:

- Breathe in deeply through the nose for a count of four....
- Hold for a count of four.
- Exhale slowly through the nose or pursed lips for a count of six. This keeps the lungs expanded longer for better oxygenation. Some preliminary research also shows that humming while exhaling relaxes the lungs even more.
- Show your child how to put her hand on her belly and feel it getting bigger and smaller with each breath.

Teach your child to start this exercise the first moment she feels a respiratory allergy coming on. Waiting until the wheezing has begun may make it more difficult to take a deep, relaxed nasal breath, which could worsen the worry and worsen the asthma.

Create Positive and Personal Tools

Allergic disorders are hard enough to live with; kids don't need a "downer" talk when they come into the office. When we see a parent and child for consultation, we start with a positive premise: "The tools your children will learn while healing their allergies will become health tools that will prevent and heal them of many other illnesses as adults. By following our allergy-alleviating prescription, your children will not only enjoy less itchy skin, a less drippy nose and wheezing lungs, and a less sensitive gut, they will also enjoy a smarter brain, a healthier heart, stronger muscles and joints, and steadier moods."

Twelve-year-old Jason came to the office for consultation with Dr. Bill to heal his allergies. After discussing the allergies, Dr.

Bill asked him what other wishes he had. First, Jason wanted to be a better soccer player. Then he revealed his worry about being so short. Aha! A teachable moment. "So, Jason, how about we put you on our Play Better Soccer Program?" He liked that. "And I'll give you a list of 'tall foods.' This program will also lessen your allergies," Dr. Bill added. After a high five, out came the "prescription pad," which you will soon read.

A few weeks later, Jason's mom called the office to deliver a happy report. "Dr. Bill, what on earth did you say to Jason? He's now doing and eating what I've been telling him for years." For Jason, and many children just like him, we make his therapeutic program relevant to his wishes.

EXERCISE YOUR ALLERGIES AWAY

While many modern lifestyle and environmental triggers are causing the rising epidemic of allergies, could this epidemic be another unhealthful effect of the sitting disease, the newest illness in the doctor's dictionary? While it's certainly not the only cause, we believe lack of movement is a major contributor to the allergy epidemic. A parallel is the rising epidemic of ADHD. Once schools had fewer recesses, more Ritalin was prescribed. Any correlation? We believe so. Children who move more often handle their allergies better, whereas excess belly fat can aggravate allergies. In our medical practice, instead of the wimpy word *overweight,* we use the more motivating term *prediabetic.* Every overweight person is by medical definition prediabetic. For those parents who still don't get shocked into action, we use the word *pre-Alzheimer's.* Let's do what we can to keep these two epidemics from developing from the *pre* stage into the full-blown versions.

Drop Excess Weight and Reduce Inflammation

Excess abdominal fat cells, known as adipocytes, dump inflammatory chemicals into the bloodstream. These chemicals knock the immune system out of balance, making you wheeze, drip, itch, and hurt. All of this compromises the health of your body's organs, but it particularly affects the lungs and joints.

In the lungs, excess fat makes already restricted breathing even more difficult. It restricts expansion of the abdomen and requires more work to breathe. Fat accumulates in the back of the throat, further narrowing the airway, which contributes to obstructive sleep apnea. Poor sleep leads to further immune system imbalance. We have noticed that once our asthmatic patients get leaner, their breathing gets easier, they sleep better, and their health improves.

Inflammatory chemicals also irritate the joints. Sore joints and bodily aches and pains mean less movement and more time sitting, which leads to even more excess body fat and more allergies. It's a vicious cycle. We encourage our patients to begin with low-impact exercise and gradually expand into an active lifestyle to get their joints back into shape.

FOCUS ON LEAN WAIST SIZE, NOT WEIGHT LOSS

The first antiallergy instruction we often prescribe for prediabetic kids is to maintain the same belt or jean size for the next two years. In our weight-control program, better thought of as a "waist" control program, we seldom ask kids to lose weight. Kids are growing so fast that if they stay the same weight and waist size for a year or two, they will naturally lean out. In our practice, *lean* doesn't necessarily mean thin. Lean means having the right weight and waist size for your individual body type. And our acronym LEAN stands for Lifestyle, Exercise, Attitude, Nutrition— the four pillars of optimal health. For more about our online LEAN program and how to become a certified LEAN coach, see www.DrSearsWellnessInstitute.org.

Improve Blood Vessels Through Movement

Each organ is only as healthy as the blood vessels that supply it. This is especially true of lungs that are affected by asthma. The lung tissue of people with asthma is often compromised, which lessens oxygenation. That's one of the reasons children with severe respiratory allergies tire easily during exercise. But movement allows lung tissues to make more tiny blood vessels called capillaries. Building extra networks of capillaries helps compensate for this lack of oxygen transfer by making more blood flow around the air sacs, called alveoli. Alveoli are like millions of tiny balloons that fill with air as you take a breath, allowing more oxygen into your body.

Movement Boosts the Body's Natural Anti-inflammatories

Nobel Prize–winning research has revealed that we have a giant personal pharmacy inside our bodies that can make most of the antiallergy medicines we need. You may ask, "Where in my body is my personal pharmacy? What medicine does it make, and how do I access it?" Let's take a trip inside the body to see what this research has taught us:

First off, think of your blood vessels as rivers and creeks. When you dump garbage in rivers, the water gets muddy and dirty, and the garbage is sticky and piles up in clumps on the banks of the river. Junk food does the same thing in our blood vessels. It makes the blood flow more slowly so that you don't get enough energy in your body to think smartly and perform well. Put in kids' terms, you don't run as fast, kick the ball as far, or dance as gracefully. Kids get the correlation: You put sticky stuff (junk food) in your mouth, you get sticky stuff in your blood, and that slows you down.

Now look at the arteries of families who eat "grow foods," like fruits, veggies, fish, greens, and beans. The blood is clean and flows through vessels like fresh water down a brand-new water slide. Once your family understands the concept of how grow foods create smooth arteries and junk food dumps sticky stuff, like pollution, into these "rivers," you can move on to the next lesson about personal pharmacies.

The lining of the blood vessels has millions of glands, like tiny squirt bottles. These are the glands that make up your own personal pharmacy. They produce natural anti-inflammatory and antiallergy medicines from your body's own chemistry set that squirt into the rivers of your bloodstream. But if your diet is filled with unhealthy food, sticky stuff piles up on the lids of these tiny squirt bottles so they can't open and release their healing fluids.

Movement will help release these natural medicines. When we run, dance, or play outside, the blood flows faster across these glands and opens the lids on these squirt bottles, letting more medicine out to heal allergies and inflammation. It's yet another reason why exercise is good for the body and for your allergies.

As you can see, lifestyle, attitude, and exercise are all important in the war against allergies and inflammation. But you are about to learn that the most significant impact you can have on your immune health involves your diet.

NUTRITIONAL CHANGES THAT HEAL ALLERGIC DISORDERS

The anti-inflammatory diet that we hope you will follow with your family is one we have used in our medical practice for the past twenty years. The term *diet* implies weight loss, but that isn't our goal. To us, the word *diet* simply means a way of eating; in truth, we're all on a diet.

How does food affect allergies? As you learned earlier, an increasingly favored term for allergies is immune system dysfunction, meaning that the immune system gets quirky and overreacts, or reacts inappropriately. We now know that the immune system is highly affected by the nutrients in food. The nutrients in food that balance the immune system are called antioxidants, and they are Mother Nature's medicines. Antioxidants give those deep colors to foods, which is why your favorite allergist, Dr. Mom, always preached: "Put more color on your plate."

The same antioxidant nutrients that provide color to a food, say the red of a tomato or the blue of a blueberry, also make these fruits and vegetables healthful. Many of the allergic *–itis* illnesses, such as arthritis, bronchitis, colitis, and dermatitis (the ABCDs), are due to the buildup of oxidants (known unaffectionately as *rust* and *wear and tear*) in the tissues. The immune system then fights this wear and tear, and sometimes overfights it, causing the skin to itch, the airways to wheeze, the joints to hurt, and the gut to be irritable. The antioxidants in the foods you will learn about in this chapter work their way into the cells of the immune system, encouraging them to behave. Think of antioxidants as providing the immune system police with the right tools to help them protect the body in the most healthful way.

The allergy-relieving nutrients in the salads, smoothies, fruits, veggies, and fish you will read about are called phytonutrients, or plant nutrients. We call them *phytos* for short. Kids can remember *phytos* much better than *antioxidants*. Here's how you can explain phytos to your kids: "When germs get into your body and cause you to wheeze or itch, it's important to feed good food to the army inside you so the army will gobble up the germs before you get sick. Fruits and veggies are 'army food.' The more fruits and veggies and seafood you feed your army, the better you'll feel." Another key to teaching nutrition to children is to make it applicable to their lives: Label these foods according to your child's favorite activity, such as *soccer foods, football foods,* or *dance foods.* Instead of *healthy foods,* call them *grow foods.*

A newly recognized area of nutritional research, called nutragenetics, studies how we can turn our allergy genes on or off with what we eat. For example, if your child is born with an asthma gene, there is a gene somewhere on his genetic code that increases the sensitivity of his lungs to pollen. That gene will always be there, and you can't take it away. The good news, and the basis behind this exciting new science of nutragenetics, is that food can affect how this gene is expressed. Imagine that the genes for asthma have an On and Off switch. Certain foods can press the Off switch, lessening the genetic tendency to wheeze. This is called turning off gene expression. If you follow our anti-inflammatory eating style, it should improve your allergies at the genetic level.

The Five-S Diet

We call the antiallergy diet we prescribe in our practice the Five-S diet, because it focuses on the following *S* foods:

Seafood: Primarily wild salmon

Smoothies: Colorful fruits and berries full of phytos

Salads: Colorful greens, vegetables, and nuts also full of phytos

Spices: Powerful anti-inflammatories

Supplements: Science-based supplements to fill nutritional gaps

Seafood

There is more science behind the use of seafood as an allergy control than there is behind any other dietary change you can make. Thus it is very important that you learn how to "go fish" as a family.

Eat fish for more color. The idea of "putting more color on your plate" not only pertains to fruits and vegetables, but also applies to seafood. Pink wild salmon are far healthier than white farmed tilapia. One day while in Alaska with Randy Hartnell, our favorite fisherman friend and owner of Vital Choice Wild Seafood & Organics, Dr. Bill asked him why salmon are so pink. Randy's answer: Imagine a salmon swimming upstream for four miles during its final marathon back to its birthplace. If kids ran uphill for four miles, they would wheeze and get short of breath, their muscles would get sore and inflamed, and their allergies would flare up all over their body. To keep this from happening to the salmon, Mother Nature provides it with a powerful antioxidant called astaxanthin, which is the nutrient that makes salmon pink. This powerful anti-inflammatory soothes the muscles in the salmon's overtaxed body. (To read more about the antiallergy and anti-inflammatory effects of astaxanthin, read *Astaxanthin: Seafood's Supernutrient,* by William Sears. Also, see VitalChoice .com for the most delicious, most nutritious, and safest seafood.)

Eat fish to breathe easier. A 2009 study from Harvard University published in the *International Archives of Allergy and Immunology* showed that teens who ate more omega-3 fatty acids (omega-3s for short) along with more fruits and vegetables had fewer symptoms of asthma and chronic bronchitis. Asthma researchers believe that this is mainly due to the anti-inflammatory effect of seafood and fruits and vegetables that help balance the immune system and lessen the sensitivity of the airways.

Eat fish to itch less. We have been writing "go fish" prescriptions in our medical practice since 1998, when hundreds of scientific articles started proving that seafood helps ease allergies. When treating eczema in particular, we focus not only on the lotions and potions you put *onto* the skin, but also the nutrients you put *into* the skin. Omega-3 fish oils are some of the most anti-inflammatory nutrients you can eat. Skin of all ages loves omega-3 oils, which help with everything from infant and childhood eczema to the inevitable "wrinkles of wisdom" in older age. Research reveals that mothers who eat more omega-3s during pregnancy have babies with less eczema. And a 2009 article in *JAMA Pediatrics* showed that early introduction of fish decreases eczema in infants.

A happy fish tale: One of our patients had a baby born with a rare genetic condition called congenital icthyosis (Greek for "fish skin"). Her skin was dry and scaly all the time. At the two-week visit, we recommended that the mother eat salmon two or three times a week and take fish oil capsules. This would allow the special fats to get into her breast milk and then into her baby's skin to help it heal. Within a month, the baby's skin was much smoother and softer, and the mother's dermatologist at UCLA was amazed. We had a very grateful mother, and a baby with healthier skin — all thanks to fish.

Eat fish to provide healthy fats for babies. The anti-inflammatory and antiallergic effects of adequate doses of omega-3s are so healing that we advise all our nursing moms to eat plenty of fish and supplement with fish oils, so that their babies get plenty of healing fats and oils through breast milk. Using new technology, we can measure the omega-3 level of mother's milk (one drop of breast milk on a test paper) and blood levels of omega-3s in infants and children (one drop of blood from a finger stick). In families with allergic disorders, this test allows us to ensure that baby is getting enough healthy fats.

Eat fish to enjoy a happy gut. A study in the *New England Journal of Medicine* showed that omega-3s can help alleviate inflammatory bowel disease, an intestinal nuisance that is affecting more and more Americans, and at a younger age. We recommend fish for all our allergy patients. And why wait until problems begin? Start making fish a routine part of an infant's diet as early as nine months of age to help *prevent* allergic and inflammatory disorders.

As you can see, there are many benefits to eating seafood—but it's important to be eating safe doses of seafood and omega-3s. Most of the omega-3 fish oil dose recommendations that you may read in older sources have recently been found to be too low. Based on the latest science about safe seafood, here are our suggestions for determining the most therapeutic dose for your child:

- For most school-age children, teens, and adults, we advise that "a gram a day keeps the allergy doctor away." This one-gram-a-day recommendation (or 1,000 milligrams) refers to the total amount of omega-3 fats; the label of every fish oil supplement lists the amount of omega-3s per serving. The two most important omega-3 fats are EPA, which provides an anti-inflammatory, or immune system balancing, effect, and DHA, which keeps cellular membranes more healthy. For reference, four ounces of sockeye salmon provides 700 to 900 milligrams of DHA/EPA. Dr. Sears's "fistful of fish" rule is that you should serve your child at least one child-sized fistful of safe seafood, preferably wild salmon, at least twice a week.
- It's best to use a fish oil that contains both DHA and EPA in a 1:1 or 2:1 ratio, which is Mother Nature's DHA/EPA ratio in wild salmon.
- For children two to five years of age, 500 milligrams of combined DHA and EPA is the recommended dose.

- For infants, we recommend about 300 milligrams of combined DHA and EPA daily. If Mom's diet includes plenty of omega-3s, her breast milk should have enough. In our medical practice, especially for our allergic families, we start salmon at seven months. A baby's brain is 60 percent fat, and the fats in salmon, like mother's milk, are the smartest fats to include in a baby's diet.

These are the *minimum* recommended dosages. Highly allergic children may need more, as recommended by your doctor.

For more information, you can Read *The Omega-3 Effect* by William Sears, Little, Brown, 2012. Here you will find the safest seafood sources, how to prepare seafood to make it tasty for your child, and more on why omega-3s work.

SAFEST SEAFOOD

In June 2013, Dr. Bill was part of a speakers' panel at GOED (Global Organization for EPA and DHA Omega 3s). The conclusion was that two fistfuls of any seafood per week is safe (that translates into 12 ounces per week for the average adult, naturally less for a child's "fistful"). Experts caution against eating too much shark, swordfish, tilefish, king mackerel, and marlin, as these may contain too much mercury.

The safest and most nutritious fish are:

Salmon, wild	Trout, freshwater
Salmon, canned	Tuna, light, canned
Anchovies	Pollack
Herring	Crab
Sardines	

Tilapia, a favorite fish on restaurant menus and fairly inexpensive in stores, is safe. However, it is one of the least nutritious fish because it has a high percentage of omega-6 oils (pro-inflammatory) and a low percentage of omega-3 oils (anti-inflammatory), the reverse of salmon.

Smoothies

How does a shake a day keep your allergies away? Again, it's all about putting more color into your mouth. Smoothies rank at the top of the list as an antiallergy prescription for these reasons:

- Children like making them and drinking them.
- They're a great way to feed your child the most colorful foods (which are the foods that contain the highest doses of phytos). You can even slip in the immune-supporting foods that your child is less fond of, such as kale or nutritional supplements.
- You can take advantage of a strong health perk called food synergy; this happens when you blend lots of colorful foods together and they enhance one another's antioxidant effects. If a smoothie could talk, it would say, "My ingredients play better as a team."
- During an asthma flare, sipping on smoothie meals over a few hours helps the gut rest while the chest uses more energy to heal. Large, solid meals can trigger heartburn and reflux, which aggravate asthma.
- The sipping solution also helps intestinal inflammation and allergies. We call this the easy-in, easy-out way of eating. Blended food exits more quickly from the stomach, is less irritating to sensitive intestinal linings, and relieves constipation.

A healthy smoothie should contain many of the ingredients listed below. Choose foods that taste good to you and feel good to your gut. Smoothies should have both protein and healthy fats, which taste better and keep you satisfied longer than a carb-rich shake. Our basic recipes follow these percentages of calories: 20 to 25 percent protein, 20 to 25 percent fats, and 50 percent carbs. Begin with smaller servings, such as a twelve-ounce shake at breakfast two to three days a week. As your body begins to crave more of this healthy start each day, you can increase the size of the shake and the frequency. Vary the fluid base and other ingredients so your taste buds can enjoy variety.

Select choices from each of these six food groups:

Healthy Fluids

- Coconut milk
- Almond milk
- Green tea
- Organic juices: green, carrot, vegetable, pomegranate

Healthy Proteins

- Organic yogurt, Greek style
- Nut butters
- Hawaiian spirulina

Healthy Protein Powder, Multi-nutrient Mix

- Juice Plus+ Complete, chocolate or vanilla, 1 scoop
- Other mixes from health food stores

Healthy Fats

- Avocados
- Nut butters
- Chia seeds, ground flaxseeds

Healthy Carbs

- Blueberries
- Strawberries
- Pomegranates
- Papayas
- Kiwifruit
- Kale
- Spinach

Special Additions

- Cinnamon
- Wheat germ
- Hawaiian spirulina
- Cacao
- Figs
- Shredded coconut
- Grated ginger

Some kids balk when you offer too much "goodness" in an adult-friendly, superhealthy smoothie. Try toning it down a bit by introducing just a basic smoothie with coconut milk (a good source of fat), naturally flavored yogurt, protein powder, banana (a great sweetener), and berries. Evolve the recipe to include more and more ingredients as your child's tastes mature.

You can see a list of smoothie recipes by searching on AskDr Sears.com.

Salads

As you're putting more color in your glass, you should also put more color on your plate. Colorful salads are superantioxidants. Dark greens and colorful vegetables work synergistically with olive oil (another powerful anti-inflammatory) to stock your child's antiallergy pharmacy with natural immune-balancing medicines. Here's an easy-reference color guide on how to fill your salad bowl. Think green and bean: kale, spinach, arugula, chard, red beans, black beans. Think red: watermelon, red peppers, tomatoes, pink grapefruit. Think yellow and orange: yellow peppers, sweet potatoes, carrots, squash. Think blue: blueberries, plums, grapes.

Begin each dinner with the salad course, before you dish up the entrée. Start this habit when the kids are young; it sends the message, "This is how our family eats dinner." Don't be too strict with hesitant kids by insisting they finish it all. Simply present small portions and model enjoyment yourself. Explain how these foods will help your child's allergies feel better. Make it fun by using chopsticks and seeing who can grab the kidney beans or sunflower seeds, or ask your toddler to pick out bites by the color (in that instance, hold the seeds!).

When our family was younger, salad used to consist of iceberg lettuce, peeled cucumbers, croutons, ranch dressing, and maybe tomatoes on a good day. Now we know there is very little value in such "junk" salads. Today, our family dinner salad has actual *green* lettuces, chopped bell peppers, nuts, seeds, raisins, dried cherries and cranberries, cucumbers (with the peel left on), tomatoes (every time), Parmesan or mozzarella cheese, and healthy olive oil–based salad dressing. Now *that's* a salad. And our kids love it!

GIVE ALLERGIC KIDS AN OIL CHANGE

Eat more	*Eat less**	*Eat none**
Fish oil	Corn oil	Hydrogenated oils
Flax oil	Soy oil	Cottonseed oil
Olive oil		
Coconut oil, virgin		
Nut oils		
Avocado oil		

* For more on why these oils can be pro-inflammatory, see *The Omega-3 Effect*, by William Sears.

Spices

Spicing up your child's diet calms down an overactive immune system. Spices that have been shown to have an immune-balancing effect are turmeric, black pepper, cinnamon, garlic, chilies, and ginger. Call them "sprinkles" as your child adds a half teaspoon of both turmeric and pepper (adding pepper increases intestinal absorption of the turmeric) to her salad or dinner and dashes cinnamon or ginger into her smoothie. Add garlic to most dinners and add chilies when you can. As you creatively market these immune-balancing foods to your children, notice how they progress from eating them only at your insistence, to liking them, and finally to craving them. This is how you turn on the wisdom of the body, as the body naturally learns to crave what is good for it.

Supplements

If we lived and ate in an ideal world where we grew our own plant foods and fished for our own seafood, we probably wouldn't need nutritional supplements. But a realistic fact of modern life is that most of us don't eat off our own farm or fish from our own ponds. And modern food processing has removed many of the nutrients from what we eat. The epidemic of immune and allergic disorders seems to parallel the developing nutritional deficiencies of our standard American diet (the SAD diet). Supplements can fill in the gaps.

We often see patients display their bag of supplements and ask us to comment on their usefulness. We usually can't, because most are not science-based. Here are the supplements we recommend in our practice, especially for our allergic patients, because they *are* science-based:

Omega-3 fish oils (see page 293 for dosages). Our favorite source of safe and nutritious salmon oil is VitalChoice.com. Cod liver oil is another healthy option. Concentrated fish oils made from small fish, such as anchovies and sardines, are also a good choice. See pages 293 and 294 for dosing. Check out DrBobsDaily.com for more information.

Fruit, vegetable, and berry supplements. If your child does not consistently eat ten servings (ten child-size fistfuls) of combined fruits and vegetables daily, which few children do, a daily supplement is needed. The one we recommend in our medical practice, and the one most supported by science, is Juice Plus+, a concentrate of twenty-five fruits, vegetables, and berries in capsule or chewable form. Health food stores also sell a variety of fruit, veggie, and berry blends in liquid, powder, chewable, and capsule form that are a healthy addition to your family's supplements (although many haven't been scientifically studied to prove they are beneficial). If your child refuses to take a kid-friendly version of the supplement, sprinkle one or two adult capsules on cereal, on a salad, or into a smoothie.

Vitamin D. Allergy doctors are giving more importance to vitamin D for balancing a quirky immune system. Numerous research studies have demonstrated that low vitamin D levels during pregnancy and infancy increase the risk of allergic disorders. Many health care practitioners are now recommending higher vitamin D supplementation during pregnancy than what is currently found in prenatal vitamins. As part of the allergy panel of blood tests, your doctor may measure your vitamin D level. As a general guide, you or your child will need to take 100 IU (international units) of vitamin D per day for every point by which you need to raise the level to a healthy range (which is between 60 and 100 nanograms per milliliter, or ng/ml). For example, if the blood test reads a level of 30 ng/ml, a daily dose of about 3,000 IU would be needed to raise it to 60 ng/ml (a rise in 30 points, multiplied by 100 IU). Again, you can turn to fish: six ounces of salmon will provide around 4,000 IU of vitamin D. Another general rule of thumb for vitamin D dosing is to take about 1,000 IU for every twenty-five pounds of body weight; this would equate to about 1,000 IU daily for infants and toddlers, 2,000 IU for school-age kids, and as much as 5,000 IU (or higher with a doctor's guidance) for teens and adults. We advise that you also check with your health care provider for dosing specific to your needs. More information is available at DrBobsDaily.com.

Probiotics. These supplements are an important step for putting better bugs in your allergic gut. As you've already learned, these "good bacteria" are residents that naturally live in the gut. In return for a nice place to live, they help regulate intestinal immunity. In kid-friendly lingo, probiotics plant a healthy garden (called flora) in your gut. Not only do these friendly and healthful bacteria talk with the immune and nervous system within the gut, but these lovely little bugs also communicate with the brain to help regulate behavior and central nervous system function.

New research is further validating the argument that what enters your mouth affects your brain and immune system. For decades, pediatric research has proven that breastfed newborns, especially premature babies, who receive their mother's milk (which is real food that contains the right intestinal bacteria) are more likely not only to grow up smarter, but also to have a healthier immune balance, with fewer –*itis* illnesses such as allergies and eczema. A day's worth (one quart) of mother's milk can nourish a baby's gut with ten trillion resident gut bacteria.

As you learned at the start of this chapter, infants who are born naturally, are breastfed, and have no antibiotic exposure should have healthy gut flora and shouldn't need routine probiotic supplementation. Infants with colic, allergies, or digestive problems may benefit from probiotics, as may children and adults with allergic or intestinal disorders and anyone who takes antibiotics. Here are some key suggestions in choosing a probiotic:

- Look for specific species. Several well-researched bacterial species have been shown to benefit intestinal and allergic disorders. These include *Lactobacillus reuteri, Lactobacillus rhamnosus* (also known as *Lactobacillus GG,* the GG referring to the last names of the two researchers who patented it), *Lactobacillus acidophilus,* and other *Lactobacillus* species. *Bifidobacterium* species have also had positive research results, as has *Streptococcus thermophilus*. A species of yeast, called *Saccharomyces boulardii,* has also been shown to help eliminate unhealthy intestinal germs and support the intestinal immune system. This yeast species can be administered alone or in conjunction with other probiotics.

- Look for multiple species. The best choice in probiotics is one that includes several strains of both *Lactobacillus* species and *Bifidobacterium* species. These will be listed on the label.

- Prebiotics. This is a fairly new concept, and it has some importance. *Pre*biotics are nondigestible fiber foods that feed the *pro*biotic bacteria and promote their growth. The two most common are inulin and oligosaccharides. Choose a probiotic that includes prebiotics on the label.

- Dosing. Follow the dosing instructions on the label. For most probiotics, suggested dosing will be in terms of "billions" of organisms per day. A typical dose ranges between one and twenty billion. For those with more complicated allergic or intestinal disorders, doses of a hundred billion or more each day may be suitable under the care of a physician. When probiotics or probiotic foods are first introduced into a gut overloaded with yeast and unhealthy bacteria, some people will experience worsened intestinal symptoms (pain, bloating, diarrhea) as the bad germs initially die off. Stop the supplement and consult with your health care provider if this occurs. You may need to reintroduce the probiotics more gradually to allow the body to adjust.

The medical research community is now taking a more serious look at probiotics and how they influence intestinal, immune, and neurologic health. Hundreds of research studies have been done so far. Even the National Institutes of Health has embarked on the Human Microbiome Project to closely examine the world of healthy bacteria that live in our bodies. This ongoing research will lead to a greater understanding of how we can live healthier, disease-free lives by focusing on gut health.

MORE ADVANCED NUTRITIONAL AND HOLISTIC APPROACHES FOR CHALLENGING ALLERGIC DISORDERS

Many allergic problems will improve or resolve with the prescribed lifestyle, exercise, attitude, and nutritional changes described so far in this chapter, along with the specific steps detailed in earlier chapters, followed in consultation with an allergy specialist. But for some families, allergic disorders pose a unique challenge that may not fully respond to this comprehensive care. Don't despair. There is still hope, and this last section offers some cutting-edge nutritional ideas that may finally provide healing.

The healing techniques we discuss in this section fall under an approach to health care called integrative medicine. This is an emerging field of practice in which classically trained physicians (like us) integrate standard medicine with alternative medical techniques. Integrative medicine involves a growing number of doctors who collaborate on their experiences and reach consensus as to which alternative medicines seem to work well. While many of these alternative medical treatments are based on sound scientific principles, they are not yet backed by large-scale research studies to prove just how effective they are. This is why most doctors are selective about some of these treatments.

As a medical family, we Sears doctors like to provide science-based advice. But allergic disorders continue to rise despite medicine's best attempts to treat and prevent them, and standard medical treatments alone don't work adequately for everyone. That is why we now explore integrative medical techniques that are well accepted among like-minded physicians, and this section provides insights into these ideas.

Low-Carb Lifestyle

As you've already learned, a healthy intestinal immune system is one aspect of achieving wellness. And for some, it is *the most important* factor in healing an allergic disorder. Helping your good probiotic gut germs thrive is the key. To best achieve this, you have to starve the unhealthy germs by depriving them of the nutrients that help them grow. Which nutrients help feed the unhealthy germs? Carbohydrates. A low-carb diet may be the most valuable healing step in hard-to-solve allergies. We have seen countless numbers of patients with chronic intestinal problems, eczema, asthma, and behavioral disorders who have improved with such diets. And we aren't the only ones — many other doctors are reporting and writing books on low-carb diets and their healing effects.

Instead of calling these diets low-carb, we prefer to use the term *right carbs*. We all need some carbs — we just have to make sure we are eating healthy carbs that will feed our bodies without feeding the bad germs in our gut.

Going right-carb is particularly important for those who try the gluten-free diet. Early books and articles written about gluten focused heavily on finding replacement foods to satisfy our craving for bread and pasta. Most advice was to eat foods loaded with carbs made from starches like rice and potatoes. Now the most current books and articles very wisely advise us to avoid carb overload across the board in order to see the best results. And as the body heals, certain carbs can be introduced later.

There are many right-carb diets to choose from; we don't have a favorite one, but we will provide a brief explanation of three lifestyles with which we have the most experience. (We prefer to call them lifestyle changes rather than diets.) To correctly follow these lifestyle changes, you must seek out a book and/or website that is dedicated to providing a complete educational presentation of everything you need to know. You should consult with your doctor and nutritionist as you begin these programs, and seek their advice on other low-carb diets that may be best suited to your unique needs. For a list of "right carbs" versus "wrong carbs," see our book *The Healthiest Kid in the Neighborhood: Ten Ways to Get Your Family on the Right Nutritional Track,* Little, Brown, 2006.

One common theme of these diets is the critical importance of avoiding food that is processed. Food should be bought fresh, in the form in which it is found in nature, and should be prepared at home. In a nutshell, an immune-balancing diet is simply a *real-food* diet. While this isn't easy to stick to in our modern society, it is an important step for those with severe allergic disorders. The good news about these eating lifestyles is that, for many, they are *temporary*. Once the gut heals and allergies subside, the principle of moderation becomes your mantra and you can learn what your family can tolerate without triggering reactions. Some will find that their problems return when they stray from the diet, and a lifelong commitment to a right-carb, real-food lifestyle is necessary. The Five-S diet we described earlier in this chapter is the most simple version of a right-carb diet. Here are some choices that take it a step further:

Paleolithic diet. The "paleo" style of eating essentially eliminates all grains, all milk products, and many starches. This is the approach I followed in addition to going gluten-free, which resulted in additional improvements in my asthma. This is also our favorite one to discuss with kids in our practice because we can explain it this way: "You get to eat like you are a caveman (or -woman). You can eat anything you could catch if you were hunting or fishing (meat, poultry, and fish). You can enjoy foods that you can pick off bushes (berries), gather in the forest (nuts and seeds), pull out of the ground (veggies), or climb up trees to reach (fruit). You can sneak eggs from chickens. But you don't own a farm, so you can't grow crops to eat (no grains, rice, or potatoes). You don't own any farm animals to eat (they must be hunted in the wild), so you can't milk cows to get milk or make cheese and yogurt." When it's presented this way, kids are more likely to embrace the change. Focus on the fun, natural foods that your cave-family *can* eat. Reflect on favorite foods that are not on the menu anymore, but reassure your child that you will enjoy them again someday when you are healthier and your allergies are gone.

Specific carbohydrate diet. Dubbed SCD, this approach involves eliminating the larger carbohydrates (such as processed fruits, starchy vegetables, all grains, processed meats, and most types of milk), which don't fully digest in most people and act as a nutrition source for intestinal yeast and unhealthy bacteria. This diet was developed several decades ago for people with inflammatory bowel disease as a way to reduce inflammation. More recently, it has been recommended for children with developmental delays as a way to eliminate intestinal yeast and bacterial overgrowth and heal a "leaky gut" (see page 158), problems that are common in those with developmental disorders. Since intestinal yeast, bacterial overgrowth, and leaky gut are major factors in allergic disorders, SCD also applies here. This diet provides clear guidance on what carbs to avoid and how to replace them with healthier, more easily digested carbs, like fresh or frozen fruits and vegetables, meats, fish, eggs, some cheese, yogurt, raw nuts, and some healthy juices. As the gut heals and healthy probiotic germs thrive, allergic symptoms may subside. One aspect of SCD that sets it apart from the paleo diet is that it allows some low-lactose natural dairy products, which are likely okay for those who don't have a specific milk protein allergy.

Gut and psychology syndrome diet. The GAPS diet follows the same basic principles as SCD. It is intended for those who suffer from mood disorders, behavioral problems, and neurodevelopmental delays as a possible manifestation of their underlying food allergies, sensitivities, and gastrointestinal problems. A primary goal of GAPS is to use the power of natural foods to heal a "leaky gut" and restore a healthy intestinal system. What sets this diet apart is that it takes a more precise step-by-step approach through several stages, gradually reintroducing more and more foods that are designed to achieve gut healing.

Which diet is right for your family? We advise the Five-S or paleo lifestyle for families with moderate allergic disorders that don't seem to involve chronic intestinal symptoms, behavioral challenges, and neurodevelopmental delays. This is the easiest diet for an entire family to follow together; even those without allergies will enjoy a "leaner" and healthier body.

If chronic intestinal symptoms are part of your allergic syndrome, SCD is a better choice for you because it focuses more on gut healing. This diet has many decades of experience behind it, and it is the one we have seen help the most people so far, including children with neurodevelopmental and behavioral disorders.

The GAPS diet is a newer approach, and it is more complicated. But its principles are sound. Those who suffer from chronic allergies accompanied by intestinal problems and mood/behavioral disorders require a more complex and whole-body approach to healing. We have seen some good results in patients so far, and we will continue to study the efficacy of the GAPS approach in the coming years.

Other well-known intestinal-healing diets include Atkins, FODMAPs, and Body Ecology.

Resources for special diets. Whichever nutritional lifestyle approach you choose, please don't try it without consulting a resource dedicated to that specific diet. This book is an introduction, but be sure to consult the following resources:

- Paleo—There are too many good books on this topic to single one out. You will find plenty to choose from online and in bookstores. We have not found a complete online guide to this diet, but you will find some useful introductory and recipe websites as you search.
- SCD—The best book on this topic is *Breaking the Vicious Cycle* by Elaine Gottschall; this is a must-read for those who want to do the diet correctly. Websites include Breaking theViciousCycle.info and PecanBread.com.
- GAPS—*Gut and Psychology Syndrome* by Natasha Campbell-McBride, MD, is the primary guide for this approach. Several commercial websites can be found by searching online.

- Overall guide to multiple special diets. The most thorough research-based guide we have found if you want a good overview of *many* special diets, with enough specific information to get started on each, is *Nourishing Hope for Autism* by Julie Matthews, CNC.

Fermented Foods: Restoring Intestinal Probiotics Naturally

Taking supplemental probiotics is one way to rebuild your gut flora. However, these bacteria are grown in a laboratory; processed; put into a capsule, powder, or liquid; and expected to grow and thrive in our body after being ingested. While research has demonstrated that these do work, a more natural way to ingest healthy germs is through foods that are rich in probiotics. A primary feature of the SCD and GAPS styles of eating is the incorporation of these foods into their protocols.

Yogurt is the classic example. Yogurt is made by a natural fermentation process involving healthy bacteria, and these healthy bacteria are present in the final product. You will see yogurt labels that state that the product contains "live active cultures." However, most store-bought yogurts don't contain enough probiotics to be therapeutic. Homemade yogurt made from fresh, raw, organic cow's milk or goat milk contains considerably more, and this is one of the best ways to achieve an adequate amount of probiotics in the diet. Also, goat milk contains more easily digestible fat and protein than cow's milk, a perk for children and adults who have intestinal allergies or food intolerances. Many other healthy fermented, probiotic foods that you can buy or make yourself may also benefit your family's gut, including:

- Kefir made from milk
- Coconut kefir (a great source of probiotics for those who are too milk-sensitive)
- Homemade sour cream (typically called crème fraîche)

- Sauerkraut and other cultured vegetables like kimchi (a Korean dish) and pickles
- Kombucha (a drink made by fermenting tea)

Detailed instructions on how to make these products are beyond the scope of this book. Most health food grocery stores carry some options. Numerous online resources are available, and the SCD and GAPS protocols provide detailed instructions on homemade yogurt, kefir, and crème fraîche. We cannot emphasize these foods enough, as we have seen many patients with chronic allergies and intestinal problems finally achieve healing when fermented foods are incorporated into their lifestyle.

One minor note: fermented foods tend to be high in histamines. Almost everyone digests these without any difficulty, even those with allergies. There is a rare condition called histamine intolerance, discussed on page 220, which results in allergic reactions to histamine foods. Watch for allergic symptoms when first introducing these fermented foods, and talk to your doctor if you believe you are reacting.

FECAL MICROBIOTA TRANSPLANT

FMT is an emerging area of research that, at first hearing, sounds absurd and extreme. But preliminary studies in mainstream medicine have shown that FMT has great efficacy in resolving chronic *Clostridium difficile* intestinal infections (severe intestinal infections triggered by certain antibiotics), inflammatory bowel disease, irritable bowel syndrome, and chronic constipation. Although these aren't the classic allergic disorders that affect most Americans, these severe intestinal conditions can be quite debilitating and can cause lifelong complications. Researchers

(continued)

have concluded that achieving a healthy gut probiotic environment is a crucial factor in these disorders, and the best way to do this is to transplant the population of fecal germs (called the microbiota) from a healthy donor. This is achieved in various ways, including enema, colonoscopy, or infusion through a long feeding tube past the stomach directly into the upper intestines. These germs repopulate the recipient's colon and bring the intestinal immune system back into balance. In some cases, this treatment is a long-term cure for what used to be considered lifelong intestinal disorders. FMT is not yet available to the general public, but if ongoing research continues to show good results, it may become routine for those who need it. This concept highlights the amazing healing properties of a healthy gut environment.

Natural Anti-inflammatory and Antiallergy Supplements

Throughout this book we have highlighted natural remedies that are specific to certain allergies. This section will focus on therapies that help balance the immune system in a way that can benefit allergic disorders in general. The efficacy of omega-3 fish oils, fruits and vegetables, vitamin D, and probiotics is well supported by research, and they are all routinely recommended by allergy specialists. Several additional nutrients that are popular among integrative and alternative health care practitioners may also have merit. But these remedies don't yet have the backing of the medical and scientific community, so you won't hear about them from a regular physician. Integrative medical practitioners, on the other hand, are well versed in their use, and we have seen some good results in families with challenging allergies in our practice. While it is better to try these under the care of a physician, you may safely begin these treatments on your own as long as you don't exceed the suggested dosing for any supplement:

Vitamins A, C, and E and zinc. These three vitamins and one mineral each play an important role in immune health and balance. Routine supplementation at the recommended daily allowance (RDA) is important to start. Simply follow the suggested dosing on the bottle. Many people, however, will benefit from the antioxidant and immune-boosting effects of higher dosing. But if doses are too high, these vitamins can be unhealthy, so high dosing should be done only under the guidance of a physician or nutritional specialist.

Pycnogenol. This nutrient is a pine bark extract and is categorized as a plant tannin. Tannins are powerful antioxidants, and they help balance the function of some immune cells. There is some research that supports the use of Pycnogenol, though not enough for it to become a mainstream therapy for allergies yet. However, it is a popular and safe nutrient for those with persistent allergic problems.

Quercetin. This is a natural pigment molecule found in fruits, vegetables, and plants. Numerous medical studies have been done that demonstrate its anti-inflammatory and antihistamine properties and its benefits in treating asthma and eczema. The research is not sufficient to satisfy mainstream medicine just yet, but it looks promising and should be considered an option.

Other herbal remedies. The field of naturopathic medicine offers some promising herbal remedies for allergies, asthma, and inflammation. Most remedies are backed by some research that demonstrates efficacy, though not enough to satisfy mainstream medicine policy makers. Commonly used herbs include stinging nettles, butterbur, lobelia, and mushrooms like cordyceps and reishi. Chinese licorice root and other herbal remedies used in traditional Chinese medicine have been shown to help with asthma symptoms. More information can be found on naturopathic websites, in books, or by consulting with a naturopathic physician. Just as regular medications should be monitored by a doctor, herbal treatments should not be taken on a long-term basis without consulting a naturopathic physician, as they can cause negative, and in some cases harmful, side effects.

I found some relief from nasal allergies by drinking a daily cup of tea made with cordyceps mushrooms; it didn't work as well as my antihistamine medication, but it did help.

Raw, local honey. Raw honey produced by your local bee population contains many of the pollens in your specific location. Some research shows that eating this honey helps desensitize the immune system to local pollen and can prevent nasal allergy and asthma flare-ups for those with seasonal allergies to pollen. Some research has not shown such a benefit, however, so the efficacy is uncertain. It is worth trying, if other measures to prevent seasonal allergy symptoms have failed. Do not give honey to infants under one year of age, as it can cause infant botulism.

Transfer factor. This is a molecule secreted by white blood cells. It helps balance the immune system by boosting the Th1 branch (the germ-fighting side) and calming down the Th2 allergic branch. It is present in colostrum and breast milk and plays an important role in establishing and maintaining a healthy immune system. As a supplement, transfer factor is extracted from either animal colostrum (milk) or eggs. In theory, it may be helpful, and science should provide clearer details in time.

Homeopathic remedies. The field of homeopathic medicine is useful and, in our experience, legitimate. It won't work for everybody, but some will find much-needed relief. The most effective way to make use of homeopathy is to visit a homeopathic physician for individualized therapy designed specifically for your body type and metabolism. We encourage our patients to explore homeopathy when traditional methods have not been adequately successful.

Homeopathic remedies are also safe to try without the guidance of an expert. I happened to find a homeopathic seasonal allergy spray very effective for my seasonal nasal allergy symptoms (made specifically for the region where I live), along with a dust allergy spray for my reactions to dust; homeopathic eye drops have also worked well for red, irritated eyes (even for conjunctivitis) in my family.

Methylation nutrients: folate and vitamin B12. Genetically inherited methylation problems are a growing problem in our society, and methylation therapy is an emerging aspect of integrative medicine. Methylation refers to the way our cells turn genes on and off, make proteins and antioxidants, and detoxify the body. It was initially applied to children with autism spectrum disorder as a way to improve immune and neurological function, and it can also alleviate allergic disorders by improving detoxification of the chemicals and toxins that may make allergies worse and by improving antioxidant function within cells. A new study published in 2014 showed that increased methylation of the ADRB2 gene (known to be involved in asthma) reduces the severity of asthma symptoms. By supplementing with the nutrients necessary for methylation metabolism, the cells (and the whole body) can better regulate DNA function so that every cell in the body works better. Managing these vitamins is best done under the care of a medical professional familiar with their use. However, you can safely use over-the-counter preparations and follow the suggested dosing.

Genetic and metabolic blood testing for methylation defects is available and is useful for those with medical insurance if it is covered. For those without coverage, testing is probably not worth the cost and may not be necessary, for two reasons: (1) over half of our population is estimated to have some degree of methylation problems, and (2) those who don't may still benefit from the folate and B12 in methyl form.

Supplementing with methylation nutrients involves the following:

- Methylfolate. Regular folic acid (found in most vitamins) isn't readily usable by people with methylation problems. *Methyl*folate, on the other hand, is taken up and used by the cells more easily so that methylation metabolism can work optimally. There are several forms of folate that work well, including methylfolate, tetrahydrofolate, and folinic acid. Look for these in multivitamins or sold as individual supplements. Follow the suggested dosing on the bottle, which is typically 200 micrograms twice daily for kids and 400 micrograms twice daily for teens and adults. Some experts advise 800 micrograms twice daily.
- Methyl B12. Vitamin B12 is also an integral part of the methylation process in the cells. Most vitamin products contain the *cyano* form of B12. But the *methyl* form is better for methylation function and is available in a growing number of over-the-counter formulations. Methyl B12 is typically dosed at several times the RDA level in order to be effective. Under the care of a doctor, some may benefit from even higher dosing, such as 1,000 micrograms daily for children and 5,000 micrograms daily for teens and adults.

Visit DrBobsDaily.com for a complete discussion on methylation supplements, probiotics, fish oil supplements, and other vitamins, minerals, and nutrients.

Holistic Hands-On Medical Therapies

Nontraditional approaches to healing chronic conditions are used by a growing number of Americans. In regard to allergic disorders, the three most common alternative approaches are acupuncture, chiropractic care, and applied kinesiology (aka muscle testing or NAET therapy).

Acupuncture. Although acupuncture sounds scary to those who are unfamiliar with it, it is backed up by some very promising research that shows efficacy, particularly for asthma and severe allergy symptoms. Acupressure may also help. Some traditional allergy specialists even incorporate acupuncture into their practice. We routinely advise our toughest cases to explore this approach.

Chiropractic. We also support the theory of chiropractic care for back pain, headaches, and other neuromuscular problems, and I visit my chiropractor several times each year. Although we don't personally witness much help with allergic disorders, we have heard many anecdotes from patients who believe they've benefitted from this care.

NAET. This alternative approach to allergy testing was introduced on page 26. Nambudripad's Allergy Elimination Technique is also used to try to make the immune system tolerant of allergens so that sufferers can resume eating allergic foods and tolerate airborne allergens. Dr. Nambudripad has provided training to many holistic practitioners nationwide to make this therapy widely available. Despite its popularity and the anecdotal positive feedback we've heard from dozens of patients, we have a difficult time wrapping our medical minds around the theory that hands-on touch therapy can influence the immune and nervous system enough to induce immune tolerance to allergens. But we are open-minded and encourage our patients to explore this option when other methods fail.

Choosing the right natural solutions to your family's allergic disorders isn't an easy task. It involves a significant investment of both time and money to explore these options. We have provided you with many choices to consider, and we have highlighted the ones we believe have the most merit. The one thing you don't have to worry about is safety; the nutritional changes, supplements, and holistic therapies described here can be considered without worry about causing harm or making allergies worse. The only downsides are the time and money spent on trying something that ultimately may not work. In consultation with your doctor and other open-minded health care practitioners, we hope you find effective solutions so that you and your children can enjoy a lifetime of health and happiness—allergy-free.

Acknowledgments

This book would not be possible without the hard work and dedication of our publisher, Little, Brown and Company. Thanks, as always, to Tracy Behar for her masterfully brilliant editing. Thanks to Terry Adams, as well, for many years of guidance. Finally, a special thanks to Denise Marcil, our agent and friend, whose expertise has been invaluable from the very beginning. And thank you to Julie Matthews, CNC, for her review of our information on special diets.

We would also like to credit the following resources that were utilized in our writing: www.AAAAI.org, the website for the American Academy of Allergy, Asthma, and Immunology; www.ACAAI.org, the website for the American College of Allergy, Asthma, and Immunology; and *Manual of Allergy and Immunology,* 5th ed., by Adelman, Casale, and Corren (Philadelphia: Lippincott, Williams & Wilkins, 2012).

Index

About the Authors

Robert W. Sears, MD, FAAP, a board-certified pediatrician, is the author of *The Vaccine Book* and *The Autism Book,* and coauthor of *The Baby Book, The Portable Pediatrician,* and *Father's First Steps.* Dr. Bob, as he likes to be called by his little patients, practices full-time in Dana Point, California, where he also lives with his wife and children. He is a medical advisor for several organizations, including La Leche League International, Kaplan University Department of Health Sciences, Talk About Curing Autism, and Nourishing Hope for Autism. He is the founder of DrBobsDaily.com, where he blogs about life in the office and provides timely news stories on health, nutrition, and other topics.

William Sears, MD, FRCP, has practiced pediatrics for more than forty years. He and his wife, Martha, a registered nurse and health consultant, are the parents of eight children and the authors of more than forty books.

Fairfax Community Library
75 Hunt St.
Fairfax, VT 05454
802-849-2420

DATE DUE

NOV 1 6 2015			